Screendance

SCREENDANCE

Inscribing the Ephemeral Image

Douglas Rosenberg

OXFORD
UNIVERSITY PRESS

Oxford University Press, Inc., publishes works that further Oxford University's objective of excellence in research, scholarship, and education.

Oxford   New York
Auckland   Cape Town   Dar es Salaam   Hong Kong   Karachi
Kuala Lumpur   Madrid   Melbourne   Mexico City   Nairobi
New Delhi   Shanghai   Taipei   Toronto

With offices in
Argentina   Austria   Brazil   Chile   Czech Republic   France   Greece
Guatemala   Hungary   Italy   Japan   Poland   Portugal   Singapore
South Korea   Switzerland   Thailand   Turkey   Ukraine   Vietnam

Published by Oxford University Press, Inc.
198 Madison Avenue, New York, New York 10016
www.oup.com

Oxford is a registered trademark of Oxford University Press

Library of Congress Cataloging-in-Publication Data
Rosenberg, Douglas.
Screendance : inscribing the ephemeral image / Douglas Rosenberg.
    p. cm.
Includes bibliographical references and index.
ISBN 978-0-19-977261-2 (alk. paper) — ISBN 978-0-19-977262-9 (alk. paper)
1. Dance in motion pictures, television, etc. I. Title.
GV1779.R665   2012
792.8—dc23   2011025327

1 3 5 7 9 8 6 4 2

Printed in the United States of America

For my father and mother

CONTENTS

LIST OF ILLUSTRATIONS

ACKNOWLEDGMENTS

I began writing this book well over a decade ago. In that time, my ideas about screendance have evolved and expanded in ways I could not have foreseen. Much of this evolution is due to the growing community of artists and thinkers who have questioned my thinking and challenged my opinions at every step of the way at conferences, symposia, and festivals around the world. Whether teaching workshops in screendance, curating screenings, or teaching students in university courses, each interaction or critical juncture has brought about new and enlightening possibilities for thinking about the form.

I am grateful to the many colleagues who, over the years, have encouraged and argued with me, listened to my often-polemic conference papers, and pushed back at the general bluster and hyperbole of my earliest presentations while I located my voice in the field.

Over the many incarnations of this book, numerous colleagues and friends have been kind enough to read my chapters and offer feedback and guidance. Naomi Jackson was an early reader who marked up piles of pages with intelligent and thoughtful suggestions, and Ellen Bromberg has offered valuable comments and support along the way and has been a gracious collaborator on a number of projects. Colleagues from the Screendance Network (funded by the Arts and Humanities Research Council, UK)— Claudia Kappenberg, Marisa Zanotti, Sarah Whatley, Kyra Norman, Simon Ellis, Ann Cooper Albright and Harmony Bench—have provided valuable critique. I must thank Ann Cooper Albright especially for both her early reading of my work and for introducing me to my editor at Oxford University Press, Norm Hirschy, who has been very patient and supportive throughout this process. Mary Sutherland is a remarkably precise copy editor who has encouraged me to use fewer words and I have tried to follow her suggestion. I would also like to thank Erica Woods Tucker, Oxford's senior production editor, for her guidance on this project. Katrina McPherson, Simon Fildes, and Bob Lockyer (who suggested me for my first international jury many years ago) have also provided insight and support. Silvina Szperling, the founder and director of the Festival Internacional de Video-Danza de Buenos Aires, has been a great supporter and colleague for many years, and is a model of the kind of passion that has globalized the field. All of these colleagues mentioned have dedicated enormous energy to the field of screendance and as such have made it a viable intellectual landscape.

Allison Bloom assisted me with an early round of proofreading, and Andrea Harris helped me enormously with the editing process at an early stage, offering historical and theoretical observations that pushed me to think about ideas I may otherwise have never reached. I also want to acknowledge some of those thinkers who have consciously contributed to the discourse of the field by putting their thoughts into writing: Erin Brannigan, Sherril Dodds, Amy Greenfield, David Vaughn, and especially Sally Banes and Noël Carroll. Very early on Sally and Noël suggested that I should write a book about screendance and made persuasive arguments to that end. To say that they were gracious and supportive mentors would be a supreme understatement, but that is, in truth, the best description for their support of my work. I have learned more than I can say from them and continue to do so.

I also wish to thank Charles and Stephanie Reinhart of the American Dance Festival for their unflagging support of my work in the context of the ADF for more than twenty-five years. Stephanie especially supported my summer class in "videodance" at ADF and attended as much as she could. I will always remember her walking into class with Talley Beatty in tow, circa 1988, precisely at the moment that I was screening Maya Deren's *A Study in Choreography For Camera*, a film in which Mr. Beatty was featured. I also fondly remember sitting in the office of ADF co-director Charles Reinhart around the same time, making my pitch that ADF invest in high-end video equipment so that I could interview all of the legendary choreographers I passed on the Duke University campus each day. He said yes, and for the next ten years I spent each summer shooting hours of conversations with a virtual living index of Modern Dance history. I also want to mention Jodee Nimerichter, the current co-director of ADF, who continues to support such projects along with the screendance symposia and international screendance festival that I direct there. It is invaluable to both my research and to the field in general.

Over the years I have received funding for various periods of research from the University of Wisconsin–Madison Graduate School, the Vilas Professorship, and the UW Arts Institute, all of which have helped me to carve out time to work on this project. Research funds from the Conney Project on Jewish Arts have helped immeasurably. Additionally, institutional support came in the form of funding for the first International Symposium on Dance for the Camera at University of Wisconsin–Madison in 2000. The resonance of that event is still evident in the larger community of screendance and in my own work as well. James Steinbach at Wisconsin Public Television has been an incredible supporter of my work for many years providing co-production on numerous screendance projects that I have directed.

Numerous residencies have allowed me the creative space to think about ways to combine theory and practice. The generosity of Janice Ross at Stanford comes to mind as does that of many other hosts including Ximena Monroy in Mexico, Karen Wood in Scotland, Kuei-Chuan Yang in Taiwan, Nuria Font in Barcelona and a number of others. I am also thankful to collaborators I have had who gave me the space to put ideas into practice such as Ken James and Cynthia Adams, Sean Curran, Sally Gross, Allen and Karen Kaeja, Joe Goode, Molissa Fenley and many others. My own work for the screen has been made poetic by dancers such as David Dorfman, Lisa Race, Sue Lee, Tania Isaac, Heidi Latsky and the community of friends and neighbors who often populate the work. I must mention Chuck Newman and Kurt Lundblad who each taught me valuable lessons about the landscape of video. Michael Eckblad and Jason Bahling are former students who are now valued collaborators in my own creative process. And Marina Kelly has been my project assistant this year helping me immeasurably as I tried to stay caught up on numerous responsibilities.

I have been lucky to have had teachers who have both inspired me and showed me new and different ways to think about art, culture, and intellectual rigor. Ted Allen and Martha Allen, Doug Hall, Paul Kos, Thanos Johnson, June Watanabe, Kenneth Meade, and Linda Frye Burnham all made me see the possibilities of an art life. My colleague Laurie Beth Clark has showed me how to be a vital and productive artist working from within a university system. Bob Skloot has been a friend and mentor over the years, and the grace with which he has navigated his creative life and his academic life has been a model for me. Lorrie Moore, Patrick Rumble, Graziella Menechella, Michael Peterson and Ksenija Bilbija have provided friendship and love, invaluable to a creative life. In general, I have come to realize that I am part of a creative, spiritual, and intellectual community that has provided a wellspring of wisdom and inspiration as I have made my way to this point.

Over the last two years, I have had the good fortune to have Nathan Jandl as my project assistant on this book. His proofreading and editorial skills, along with his general intellectual curiosity and breadth of knowledge about the way good writing is created, has made it possible for me to get to the end of this process. He has, without a doubt, made me a better writer in every way and has, quite frankly, become a teacher for me. Nathan read every word I wrote and gave me invaluable feedback and suggestions as he assisted me through the final stages of this book. His contribution to the process was immeasurable.

Finally, I want to thank my partner in life, Li Chiao-Ping, an exquisite choreographer and dancer as well as my collaborator for some twenty years, and our son, Jacob, who constantly educates me in what really matters in life.

ABOUT THE COMPANION WEBSITE

www.oup.com/us/screendance

Oxford University Press has created a companion website to accompany this book. The website contains supplemental illustrations, each marked in the text with the symbol ⊜. Readers are encouraged to turn to the website whenever they see this symbol.

PREFACE

> If we compare one art to another, it is not with the intention of contrasting their
> actuality, but to speak rather of the motivations and properties such as are
> admissible to the world of verbal ideas.
>
> Mark Rothko, *The Artist's Reality: Philosophies of Art*

As an artist who also writes, I approached this project with some trepida-
tion. Artists who maintain a studio practice and simultaneously publish
critical texts in the same field often feel themselves mistrusted in both
areas of production.[1] The result of such a perception is often an *internalized*
mistrust of the ways in which we negotiate our own disciplinary boundaries. Is our artistic production subject to our own criticality as it is written
on the page or delivered as lectures in conferences and elsewhere? And how
does one negotiate the sensitive relationship between theory and practice,
practice and theory?

Further complicating the issue of artistic identity is the question of
whether one teaches in the academy. The identity of "university professor"
is a powerful fulcrum in discussions about privilege, artistic integrity, and
artistic citizenship, often earning one the label of "academic," which, while
a positive description in certain circles may be pejorative in others.
Notwithstanding recent ideas about the porosity of disciplinary boundaries, and the almost unbroken flow between the performative and the mediated in general, the firmament between practice and theory seems to be the
last bastion to fall. This is not without some irony; in both the "art" and
"dance" worlds as well as the "film" world, there is a long and important
history of practicing artists writing, so to speak, from *inside the circle*. Such
artist's writing has spoken to both producers of objects and/or visual culture, as well as receivers of that culture and an interested intellectual contingent as well. Some take the form of manifesto such as Sol Lewitt's
Sentences on Conceptual Art, Lars Von Trier's *Dogma 95*, or Yvonne Rainer's

NO Manifesto, but others contribute clear and direct theoretical and/or philosophical texts that compliment and underpin their nontextual creative output.

But perhaps the most appropriate examples for the purpose of this discussion are Maya Deren and Sergei Eisenstein. Both Deren and Eisenstein made moving images and theory at the cusp of a moment when the horizon of their respective practices was barely visible. They merged theory and practice in ways that could be seen as models for screendance artists. Even though Deren was not associated with an institute of higher education, her theoretical writings are essential reading for any filmmaker. Eisenstein, whose writings form a basis for understanding his ideas about the art of montage, taught at the Russian film school GIK, where he was charged with contributing curriculum.[2] There are numerous examples of filmmakers from Eisenstein on whose writing has occupied a portion of their creative output, including Stan Brakhage, Trinh T. Minh-ha, Jean Luc Godard, François Truffaut, and Laura Mulvey. Apart from film, the visual arts also have a number of salient examples of theorist/artists who have written philosophical or critical texts, such as Mark Rothko,[3] Donald Judd,[4] and Robert Morris.[5] And there are many examples of critic/poets across the arts, including Edwin Denby, John Ashbery, and Peter Schjeldahl, all of whom have contributed important work as producers of both "art" and critical texts. In dance we can cite choreographers as diverse as Leonid Massine, Yvonne Rainer, and Doris Humphrey as artists who sought to further articulate their ideas through the writing of texts, thus approaching the creative practice from dual overlapping points of reference. Such a model informs a contemporary turn toward a practice in which theory and production flow seamlessly into text and back to object or performance.

My own history merges practice with both writing and teaching. The circular feedback loop that is created as one engages a practice from three such points of entry encourages a very particular kind of reflexivity because one is inside the circle of makers while at the same time encircled by another ring of critical thinking. It is a liminal state in which the boundaries between producer of culture and articulator of cultural production are tidal in their ebb and flow: ideas manifest as films and other projects and often simultaneously flow into critical or theoretical musing, and creative output is split into multidisciplinary tributaries. Since the early 1980s I have maintained a visual art practice that has consistently overlapped with the practice of dance. My work in video and performance morphed into "videodance" in the late 1980s, and then into collaborative live work in the form of collaborative multi-media projects for the theater or simply "performance art," which included dancers and made use of projected and prerecorded imagery, slides, and other media. I have done a considerable amount of dance documentation with the American Dance Festival, among others, and have collaborated with countless choreographers on works made primarily for the screen as well, ultimately thinking about this work under the rubric of "screendance." As I find myself surrounded by artists in one discreet area of practice, I am always aware of the histories and theories of another complimentary practice across disciplinary boundaries. The nexus and synergy between histories and disciplines, and the *frisson* that often occurs in those overlaps, is what pushed me toward an interdisciplinary art practice and into the study of dance alongside the visual arts. That same *frisson* is what prompted me toward the intermingling of discreet areas of practice, as well as toward writing about the territories that are formed out of such layering. This book is the product of my own desire to think about screendance within ever increasing concentric circles of creative inquiry and ever widening frames of reference.

Introduction

Inscribing Hybridity

The relationship between the practice of dance and the technologies of representation is complex and interdependent. As movement migrates to the screen, live dance collides with its mediated other, resulting in new and evolving methods of inscription. This complicated and intricate duet takes place as the body in motion inscribes itself within the confines and the edges of the camera's frame: a collaborative, hybrid undertaking. The collaborators in this process of inscription are engaged in the creation of screendance, which from the outside resembles not so much the making of a dance in the traditional sense but the kind of production that takes place in a small factory or laboratory. It is less a performance than an elaborate, deconstructed photo session, unfolding temporally, frame by frame. The collaborators experiment with choreographic form as well as the formal structure of filmmaking itself, altering camera placement, shot composition, and visual space to find the most efficient and esthetic methods of framing movement. Within this conceptual shift from live to mediatized representation, the "dance" is reduced to the smallest sum of its parts.[1] A gesture is isolated and viewed for its innate characteristics, as if through a microscope, and there is a scientific precision involved in the reproduction of even fleeting sequences of movement. The site of creation moves from a *workspace* to a *workflow*, in which production is not sequential or centralized but is rather a simultaneous fabrication of disparate parts, self-contained units that will be reconfigured in the future. Dance in cinematic space is necessarily conceived as a product of individual parts, and as the screendance progresses from preproduction to production to postproduction, additional elements are constructed, added, or removed.

Like industrial production, the context of the work is largely unintelligible until the parts are assembled according to the imagination of the designer or, in the case of screendance, the director and/or choreographer.

In the construction of a screendance, the traditional linearity of the choreographic process is flayed open and exposed to a very particular kind of scrutiny. Composition may come in isolated bits; kinesthetic transitions may become virtual or nonexistent, slated to be inserted later in the editing process. Movements and gestures, released from the physical boundaries of weight, time, and space, are digitally archived to be retrieved and reconstructed at a later date. The dance/dancing thus becomes malleable, fluid, and available as a kind of digital text.

The (re)production of this dance, then, is as conceptual as it is physical, as much digital construction as corporeal performance. While the twentieth century saw great progress made in the space where dance and media overlap, including seminal films by Maya Deren, Norman McLaren, and others, postmillennial experiments in the merging of dance and media have the potential to revolutionize conventional conceptions of both dance and dance-media hybrids. Migrating dance to camera space is a process of meta-production that resembles something similar to contact improvisation—and in a sense, it *is* about both contact and improvisation.[2] One participant—the dancer—moves freely, unencumbered, while the other—the camera operator—is tethered by the camera, a prosthetic image-gathering device that by necessity becomes an extension of the body. Although the contact is often metaphorical, there is an intense relationship between the camera and the dancer, one that often begins with improvisation. In this process, numerous diversions and details vie for the eye's attention. But at the center is the body in motion: there the camera fixes its gaze. And there the camera allows for a kind of engaged looking at the body that is unique to that device. The camera functions for the director as a microscope functions for the pathologist, providing a way of seeing that is both privileged and functional, as well as an opportunity to isolate and track the smallest bits of data, often invisible in isolation but rendered poetic in their mediatized physicality.

In an era in which interdisciplinarity is greatly valued in both the arts and academe, the hybrid form of screendance offers a compelling lens for new theories and practices. In this book, I advocate for a model of screendance that not only attempts an active engagement with multiple discourses outside of the conventional narrative of dance but also reflects the inherent interdisciplinarity of screendance itself. This interdisciplinarity is partially the product of the varying tensions at play throughout the history of screendance and its inherent, inevitable hybridity: tensions between different art genres, between high and mass culture, and between the body and its own mediation. If screendance is to significantly exert its presence, it needs to establish its own historical foundation as well as a working theoretical framework and genre specificity. To the issue of history, while there have been various attempts to structure a historical timeline for screendance, such efforts have tended to reify existing paradigms, similar to the heroic mythologies that flow from modernist narratives.[3] But historiographies that trace the entire arc of screendance from its liberation from the still frame of photography through the present—and in doing so question both critical status quos and their inhered, incomplete histories—are only now being written. Moreover, until recently screendance has lacked a robust critical center from which to address the analytical and theoretical problems unique to the form.[4]

This complex dialog is reflected in the very name "screendance," and I offer a brief rationale for the choices made in regard to describing the practice and its subcategories. I have chosen the term "screendance" as the most accurate way to describe the passage of "dance," via its mediated image, to any and all screens without articulating materiality. That is to say, screendance speaks of the *end point* or the *point of reception* by the viewer and not of the material form of the production in the way that "videodance" refers to the actual production media or method of inscription. Similarly, the term "filmdance" or "cine-dance" situates the work within the historical and material culture of film. The term "dance for camera" is equally fraught, as it suggests a paradigm in which dance is privileged by virtue of its placement in the descriptive title, though also in service to the camera; further, it suggests that it is the language of dance that exercises authority over the method of its visualization. Screendance, then, though not a perfect term, implies that the method of apprehension (the screen) modifies the activity it inscribes (dance); in doing so it codifies a particular space of representation and, by extension, meaning. Those other terms—videodance, filmdance, dance for camera, and so forth—should instead be considered as specific subcategories of screendance and will be excavated further in the pages that follow.

Contextualizing screendance, of course, is not a simple matter. Screendance is an intentionally broad term that may address any and all work that includes dance *and* film or video as well as other screen-based software/hardware configurations. Yet, it is hampered by its lack of stylistic differentiations, which are found in other, evolved art forms. Such differentiations allow for critical analysis and comparison. For example, "dance," as a general term, may include ballroom, jazz, ballet, and modern, just as "art" as a general term may include impressionist painting, conceptual art, and multiple forms of sculpture. The arena in which these works are presented further contextualizes them and sets the tone for discourse and critique. Screendance, as a genre, is ill-equipped to support a discourse without such contextualization. The first step toward criticality, therefore, is to differentiate genres within the larger category, as has been done in dance and the fine arts generally. A documentary cannot be critiqued in the same way that a choreography for the camera might; an experimental work requires a completely different discourse. At the moment, within the field, there are no clear definitions or boundaries for the terminology commonly used to describe the various subcategories of screendance, resulting in a lack of clarity and slippage in regard to both meaning and context.

While screendance has articulated its outlines in the broadest strokes, enough to be considered a practice, the field currently suffers from a crisis of identity in three distinct ways. First, screendance is often aligned with dance or marginalized as a subgenre of modern dance, placed solely in the context of dance history. This type of historical repression perpetuates an incomplete reading of the histories of both dancing bodies and mediatized bodies; there we overlook or suppress the relationship between bodies in motion and moving image production, which has existed since the earliest days of film. Moreover, such a classification denies the impact of the other arts on screendance, and denies screendance a place in the larger canons of art history and practice in the modern era. Institutions, including the academy, tend to parse art practice into genres that are media-specific, although conceptual ripples often connect seemingly disparate practices to each other in ways that are not immediately readable. The very fact that screendance has always been a hybrid form instantiates a critique that disrupts many of the epistemological categories still preserved in our academies and elsewhere.

Second, although the global community of screendance has grown in both scale and artistry in recent years, bolstered by an increasingly media-savvy culture and ever more omnipresent technologies (informing not only screendance but also contemporary choreography), this community remains largely virtual, spread out over continents and electronic mailing lists, occasionally meeting at conferences or festivals. Makers of screendance typically work in isolation, shooting, editing, and screening work in darkened spaces without any audience interaction. When the work does reach an audience, viewers are further isolated from the makers because the artists are often absent from screenings, and there is no "live" performance as such. Without an organized, physical sense of community, the work seems to be in its own orbit, a closed system that lacks an external feedback loop. This lack of community is exacerbated by tangible tensions concerning issues of form and content, and of curation and spectatorship, all of which contribute to the anxiety of identity from which screendance suffers.

Recent years have witnessed an expansion of international festivals and screening venues, which helpfully build a sense of community by augmenting the discursive environment of screendance. And yet, the majority of these events, especially those that take place in the United States, focus on exposing audiences to screendance as a "new form," typically without a corresponding critical component that situates the work in historical, theoretical, or cultural contexts.[5] The result is the presentation of many exhibitions of screendance works but disproportionally little critical dialog—or there is discourse, but it is disconnected from the presentation of works. Generally this practice keeps screendance artificially confined to the festival model ("dance film festivals" or "video dance festivals") and as such delimits its relationship to the film and video communities outside of the dance world, as well as to larger discourses about art and the moving image.[6] The lack of actual curatorial activism—the lack of curators whose choices make a particular statement about the form—within the festival format in fact limits dialog between individual works and the larger history of the form.[7]

If the institutional recognition of screendance has spurred festivals and screening venues, then, it has simultaneously created a social space in which this work is herded into those subcategories that often lack curatorial clarity. Instead, these festivals often seem to be programmed for reasons that have more to do with audience-building than raising questions about the art form. Festivals need to sell tickets and fill seats, so they become by necessity more about advocacy than criticality. Programming, therefore, as opposed to rigorous, informed, or thoughtful curating, remains the norm, and festivals strive to alternate light with dark, funny with serious, to ensure that the audience is suitably engaged. Encouraging this kind of viewing diminishes the possibility of creating a site for critical and cultural inquiry by elevating issues and values more closely aligned with entertainment or marketability than critical analysis and understanding.

And finally, screendance's third crisis of identity pivots on the fact that critical dialogue or scholarship on the form has been slow to evolve within the academic community, despite the ever-expanding exhibition of new work in festivals around the world.[8] In the late twentieth century, a smattering of critical writings on screendance began to appear, often published in film journals, with the occasional appearance in a dance publication.

Considerably more discourse on screendance has been generated in recent years, in books and journals as well as international conferences and festivals. But much of this discourse relies on methodologies that are either outmoded or inadequate to the demands of the genre.[9] Again, as screendance is persistently understood through dance narratives (and particularly historical modern dance narratives), other trajectories outside of dance are overlooked or denied. Thus, many non-dance points of entry and inquiry, including those from film, video, and visual art, are lacking. Contemporary criticism across the arts employs methods derived from, among other sources, psychoanalytic, materialist, feminist, and queer modes of analysis. Yet, this sort of in-depth, critical, and interdisciplinary reading is overlooked in screendance in favor of a modernist emphasis on materiality or on a model in which dance and film are bifurcated and treated as if separate entities.

We can trace the genealogy of this bifurcation in both historical and contemporary writing on the intersection of moving images and mediated bodies by looking at some early, extant critical writing. In his 1967 essay "Cine Dance and Two Notes," the filmmaker Sydney Peterson explored the "problem of media in a composite medium, which had its own well-established hierarchy."[10] He pointed out that dance is in effect "a competing medium," resulting in the incompatibility of dance and cinema. Further, in speaking about Maya Deren's *A Study in Choreography for Camera*, Peterson attributed the success of Deren's film to her editing techniques, which he characterized as "tricks and magic" that hearken back to Georges Méliès and earlier, in which a reliance on prestidigitation supplanted film's discovery of its own "potential as a dramatic and narrative medium."[11] In fact, he suggested that artists who wish to combine dance and film might model a pre-cinematic time as far back as the seventeenth century when magical effects could be found in the theater. A similar observation underlies Jeffrey Bush and Peter Z. Grossman's 1975 argument that video comprises "a different world" from the realm of dance and that its techniques, inherited from the essentially dramatic nature of cinema, are at odds with dance's spatial and temporal elements.[12] Bush and Grossman endorse a concept of "videodance" as a "separate branch of both dance and video, with its own requirements, its own techniques, and its own aesthetic principles."[13] But even as they approach videodance as an independent, hybrid genre, much of their essay attacks television dance as inadequate to an authentic representation of live dance. Instead, they propose that dance artists must "take control of the medium for themselves" in order to mine the potential of videodance for choreographic development.[14] This statement ultimately reinforces a trope that keeps the potential for a hybrid of dance and media tethered to ideas about *choreographic* space as it exists in live, theatrical dance. This trope then ignores the possibility of new ways of thinking about choreography in the site-specificity of media space and relies on preexisting paradigms of dance as an autonomous form, not subject to disciplinary hybridization. Such paradigms insist on the respective autonomies of dance and film.

One of the first to advocate for screendance untethered to live dance or traditional dance techniques was Amy Greenfield, who, in her 1970 article "Dance as Film," argues for a model of "filmic dance."[15] In contrast to medium-specific approaches, she does not see dance and film as incompatible forms but rather as siblings with a great deal in common: "Film and dance are the only two art forms that move in both time and space. That is a strong basis on which to form a common language."[16] Greenfield points out the inevitable hybridity as dancing bodies migrate to film, and she contends that "What you perceive as 'dance motion' in the projected image is the relative coordination of many kinds of motion, and not one alone."[17] In a similar vein, the film critic and philosopher Noël Carroll posits that modernist criticism's overly exclusive stance that cine-dance can be identified by and should possess uniquely cinematic traits overlooks the fact that filmic space and time are indeed possible in other genres. Carroll sketches an ontological account of what he calls "moving-picture dance," a definition broad and inclusive enough to deal with the hybridity of the form and the evolving nature of the technologies that continually transform the medium.[18] Carroll's rigorous analytic approach, as well as his method of looking at the overlap of dance-film through other esthetic and historical lenses (such as *ballets méchaniques*), offers an instructive model of an interdisciplinary critical analysis, which includes and considers a variety of contexts and historical developments surrounding the form.[19]

An example may help illustrate the benefits of a critical landscape to an emerging field, in order to highlight the potential gains screendance stands to make if it can be turned toward increased historicity, criticality, and interdisciplinary dialog. In the 1970s and 1980s, video art was flourishing. Dedicated screening venues sprang up across the United States as video art festivals received local and national funding and support. When the National Endowment for the Arts came under increasing attack, the support for such work (work often engaged in cultural critique) quickly disappeared. Prior to the collapse of the screening circuit, however, the art form was legitimized by published critical writing and through institutional recognition, which articulated video art as a viable area of contemporary art practice. Such an index of scholarship and writing, both historical and contemporary, catalyzes a continuing critical dialog about video and its relationship to other disciplines, cultural moments, and the art world in general. Although there are no longer legions of video art festivals, scores of museums, galleries, and other venues have recognized the value of such work, and it has become a part of the twentieth-century (and beyond) canon. Video art now lives in the same house as painting, sculpture, and other traditional forms—a house that, in fact, has become quite crowded as video and video installation have become the art of the new millennium.

This brief history of video art emphasizes that proactively framing a discourse *defines the terms* of the discourse. And it suggests that the lack of theoretical discourse relating to screendance is a situation of our own making, as is the level and seriousness of the discourse that does exist. For many years I have attempted to broaden the canon of dance film and video to one that is more inclusive both in theory and in practice, and to provoke artists and critics toward into a deeper and more meaningful involvement with screendance. Such a broadening must begin with the makers of screendance, as the way that we articulate our endeavors in this field (or fail to do so) frames the discourse that follows. While the field is populated by artists who are deeply committed to the genre, *collectively* we need to address the way in which the dialog of screendance is framed and contextualized. Television or the internet, for example, are portals through which viewers may first encounter works of screendance, and both frame content very particular ways. Yet that same work is often viewed in entirely different contexts, such as galleries, festivals, and others venues that recontextualize the viewing paradigm. It seems only appropriate to ponder how that work circulates as culture within a discursive frame and how such viewing platforms alter the reception of screendance. This kind of close reading of both the work and its presentation ultimately allows for a deeper understanding of the work and, by extension, its relationship to the culture that produces and consumes it.

Screendance, though practiced with considerable vigor over the course of the last century, has always been a marginal genre. Never quite fitting within the preexisting structures of cinema or video art, it has been treated with some derision by both genres. More surprisingly perhaps, screendance has never been completely embraced by any faction within the mainstream dance community (although there have been isolated moments when screendance finds itself in favor within the larger construct of dance, either modern or postmodern). Generally, these moments of inclusion coincide with a new or evolving technology, such as film in the late nineteenth, early twentieth century in the work of Thomas Edison at his Black Maria Studio; in the 1940s and 1950s through the cine-dance work of Maya Deren, Shirley

Clarke, Norman McLaren, and others, or video in the late 1960s through the 1980s. Currently, given the availability and increased awareness of new media and digital technologies, dance again finds itself the object of much affection within the frame.

It is my intention to create a context for a specific kind of history, to provide starting points for these key areas—the evolution of historical narrative(s), establishing critical paradigms, and drawing practitioners into critical and theoretical inquiry—and to suggest certain directions such work might pursue. Chapter 1 investigates site-specificity in relation to screendance, articulating the very particular space of the camera and describing how that space inscribes content and meaning as one frames movement within the lens of the camera. Documentation is often thought of as a simple unmediated recording of an event that maintains both its original intent and temporality, but even documentation is undertheorized, and it is in no way simply an objective view of a dance event. Cameras are prosthetic devices for extending one's range of vision; however, they do not duplicate vision—they *replace* how we see the world with a mediated version of what we desire the world to look like. As such, they have the potential to add layers of artifice to the event they are meant to record. This first chapter suggests theoretical frameworks for thinking about both the differences and similarities between media as a method for archiving and also as a primary site for art making.

Chapter 2 offers a trajectory of media specificity in relation to dance on screen by tracing the evolution of dancing bodies on screen and the material by which they are inscribed. Here I discuss a body of work important to the development of screendance, offering a context for particular readings of the work in a theoretical frame. My analysis moves laterally across the art world to connect screendance practice to other significant esthetic and cultural movements. As a result, I embed the history of screendance in larger historical contexts. One of those historical contexts centers on the 1960s, in which the changes in the way that media circulated brought vastly different esthetic and theoretical concerns to bear for both artists and society in general.

An analysis or account of screendance is incomplete without looking beyond the form itself and toward shifting cultural ideas about bodies and mediation. Chapter 3 theorizes the creation of impossible or screenic bodies via screen techniques. Screendance is a literal construction of a choreography that is contingent upon its rendering in either film, video, or digital technologies. Neither the dance nor the method of rendering are in service to each other but are instead partners or collaborators in the creation of a hybrid form. It is a double graft, both screenic and kinesthetic.

Recorporealization occurs at the interstices between the multiple practices of dance and the techniques and materiality of media. It is based on the idea that the filmed body is a kind of Frankenstein, temporally dislocated and awaiting authorial reanimation.[20] The raw data of the dancing body is stitched together in the editing process of either film or video, resulting in an *impossible* body. That body is unencumbered by gravity, technique, temporal restraints, even death. The chapter also discusses how, even in death, film and digital media can resurrect the deceased body and keep its mediated self alive ad infinitum.

Chapter 4 examines the historical and cultural impact of the development of video technologies, not only as a method of recording but as a paradigmatic shift in the way that bodies are represented on screen. Video technologies introduced the immediate feedback loop—the real-time representation of self in real, architectural space, and the simultaneous apparition of self in synthetic, screenic space. Such a loop has permeated twenty-first century culture and made the screen a destination for dance in the new millennium.

Chapter 5 uses Marcel Duchamp's well-known sculpture—*The Bride Stripped Bare by Her Bachelors, Even*—as a metaphor for a particular kind of courtship, which is present throughout the history of mediated dance. This courtship, which begins with the advent of technologies for extending vision and continues through the histories of film, video, digital imaging, and beyond, is one in which the very nature of dance is contested and reconsidered.

In chapter 6 screendance is framed as a diasporic culture, constantly migrating through host cultures and assuming various vernacular elements of those cultures while often struggling to maintain its own identity. Screendance, as it passes through such host cultures, maintains the traces of each encounter in a kind of ghosting that ultimately alters the form and substance of screendance itself. It is a process of inscription that reflects the gestures of dancing bodies as well as the signifying characters of the site and other forces of production.

In chapter 7 I situate the practice of curating within a discussion of criticality and address the need for both in the field of screendance. Criticality and activist curating practices encourage an expanded notion of screendance as a viable art form. The typical models of exhibition and circulation by which screendance enters the culture is at odds with other modes of contemporary arts practices, following instead a model somewhere between film festivals and dance performances. Typically, dance is *programmed* while art is *curated*, a model that has been adopted by screendance within the festival circuit. I address the tension present in screendance as these two modes of presentation and organization confront each other.

Chapter 8 reconsiders connoisseurship and its possible relationship to screendance, focusing on spectatorship, the audience, and the role of connoisseurship, the phenomena in which literacy grows through the collaborative efforts of curators, makers, and finally audience members and patrons. Connoisseurship, as such, might be described as a desired outcome of any art form, including screendance.

Chapter 9, closes in on a theory of screendance, suggesting paradigms intended to describe observations about the field and possible approaches to amending the way we think about the practice. Subsequent to addressing ideas by the feminist film theorist Laura Mulvey, the dance historian John Martin, and the cultural critic Walter Benjamin, I offer close readings of two important works for the screen, Anne Teresa De Keersmaeker's *Rosa Danst Rosas* and Hilary Harris's *Nine Variations on a Dance Theme*, in order to point toward the way meaning is constructed via strategies of framing the body, gender, and the performative nature of editing. Both works are viewed while thinking about the camera as a carnivorous image-prosthetic device.

The tenth and concluding chapter attempts to locate the practice of screendance in academe, and in so doing maps out a new territory for pedagogy inclusive of the histories of the visual arts and other contemporary practices that have helped shape the genre. It offers a new paradigm for teaching the subject in higher education, one that relies more on the practices of the arts outside of the purview of dance while acknowledging that dance is a vital component of the framework in which screendance is placed.

Screendance promises to be an especially vital subject in the twenty-first century. We live in an era of hybridity: the merging of genres shows itself in the arts as well as in our daily lives. The work that occurs at the intersection of dance and media necessarily speaks two languages simultaneously. Screendance is possible only in the hybrid space where the lingua franca of dance and the lingua franca of the method of inscription overlap. The materiality of the recording format (film, video, or digital media) cannot be discounted nor can the choreographic language by which the work is inscribed. Each layer produces a metaphoric value quite different from another. Screendance's mediated duet with the body is especially important since the body has been the locus of so much recent theoretical work. The body, as it is mediated by technology, is at the forefront of emerging theories about identity, agency, performance, and hybridity. Screendance can indeed proactively engage this dialogue and simultaneously alter its landscape.

Doing so honors the history of the genre and those who negotiated spaces for its exploration, ensuring that the work of those who pushed the boundaries of dance and film will be more than a faint echo in that history.

In order to better understand contemporary screendance and to take advantage of the enormous potential for community among current practitioners in this and adjacent fields, it is crucial that we develop new approaches to the genre. Rather than thinking of this work as a mere circumstance of other genres, we can conceive of it as a distinct interdisciplinary development in the history of modern and postmodern art, worthy of study on its own terms. Thus, this book articulates a history of screendance that is inclusive of, and acknowledges the influence of, disparate sources—including those outside of dance. In addition, it is important to establish this history as a common history, shared by those who make or study screendance.

In order to further define screendance as a genre unto itself, we need new ways of conceptualizing the intersections between dance and its mediated image, new theories that privilege neither, and therefore embrace sources outside of both. This new theory must necessarily be both rigorous in the way in which it applies existing as well as new knowledges to screendance and interdisciplinary in its breadth. Adjunct to this theory, we must develop appropriate critical strategies for our genre that situate it in the larger discourse of art practice. Screendance studies must take into account emerging forms of representation and technologies, as well as new and historical representations of mediatized dancing bodies, while remaining fully conscious of contemporary and historical practices of the arts in general.

Screendance has its own particular history, even though that history is still in the process of inscription and is rarely recounted as a coherent narrative. Screendance has always been at the margins of moving image and dance practice, perhaps because it can either extend dance into the mainstream in mediated form, or it can create an entirely new hybrid form, a dismantling of tradition that rejects and challenges the mainstream. It is in this most marginal of spaces that outsider filmmakers like Maya Deren, Shirley Clarke, and Doris Chase carved out territory at the intersection of the moving image and the moving body, enabling them to create works seminal to the history of both screendance and independent media practice. Perhaps it was the very marginalization of the art form that enabled these experimental works, in the sense that opportunities to create outside of the established esthetic norm for women artists, proto feminists and others generally did not exist in mainstream film. In the current climate, though, as art forms—especially the less dominant ones—compete for dwindling funding, the territory that these pioneering artists claimed is dangerously close to being sacrificed for mainstream recognition and acceptance of screendance as a populist media. Conversely, the survival of screendance as a serious art form requires that we work toward developing a history, a canon, and a body of criticism (if only to create a starting point for further dialog). If screendance is consistently presented in ways disconnected to larger critical, social, and artistic concerns, it compromises its own viability as a socially, artistically, and institutionally meaningful form.

Screendance is a practice that is in constant flux. In the past, the field has made a number of attempts to define itself as other than film, video art, performance art, live dance, and any number of extant practices. However, screendance is *all* of those, as well as a hybrid of impulses from such disparate sources as the visual arts, Hollywood and literature. I propose that screendance, aside from its impulses, is an overarching genre with a multitude of subgenres. Through theorization and curation, screendance can be located within the larger frame of the visual arts with relationships to dance, film, and other sources that do not define but rather deepen the practice. This book is an attempt to initiate a theory that defines screendance, to open screendance up to further theorization, and to filter it through a set of lenses that can provide new and renewed perspectives on the form. These lenses are by no means definitive or finite; as a sampling, however, they should be understood to signify the richness and diversity of the history and practice of screendance.

CHAPTER 1

Archives and Architecture

Dance is, by its very nature, an ephemeral art form. It is also one that is constantly defining and redefining itself in relation to both dance culture and its own contemporary era. Although dance has always had at least a tangential relationship with technology, the boundaries between dance practice and the technologies of visuality have become increasingly porous since the latter part of the twentieth century. Indeed, as dance has moved into the twenty-first century, we have seen a grafting of dance and technology, which has led to a number of hybrid forms, screendance being one such form. Dances made for screens or synthetic spaces, with or without the use of a camera as a portal, flow from the embrace of technology as part of the creative process.[1] Mediated dance assumes many forms; however, the critical or analytical reading of a hybrid or grafted dance-media work is necessarily informed by all of the elements present up to and including the end point or reception site of the work. These include both form and content, as well as the social and cultural referencing made possible by postmodern philosophies and their cumulative meta-narratives. The author Sally Ann Ness notes that dance is already a "kind of writing" or "something that approximates writing." As such, the gestures contained within dance perform a type of inscription. Such inscription then, when migrated to media space, mingles with the semiotic markers consistent with that new space, and the subsequent inscription becomes even more complex.[2]

While dance is ostensibly the stimulus for a number of hybrid practices such as screendance—practices I refer to as meta-dance—it may also be that dance is the beneficiary of a particular kind of longing for kinesthetic stimulus that emerges from the space of optical media. Meta-dance is an undertaking in which choreographic movement is filtered through a complex architectural system of digital interventions and mediation, enveloping contemporary dance, altering it, and often recasting it as data in a postmodern site-specific construction. Screendance is a part of this rhizomatic movement; it is created in a *liminal* space between what is traditionally understood as "dance" and its (semi) permanent inscription as a replayable media archive. That media, be it film, video, digital technologies, or other, is a holding place or transfer point for its final end point as a screen image. Screendance therefore remains in archival limbo until the point at which it is *recorporealized* for public performance. The language by which it does this effectively frames the discourse that surrounds the screenic object.

Critical discourse relies on language (either written or spoken) to communicate knowledge about particular areas of research and, while all the terms used here to describe the work in question—"dance for the camera," "video dance," "cine-dance," "screendance,"—may seem somewhat interchangeable, they are, in actuality, quite specific. Each term speaks to a particular combination of performance and materiality, and each sites the dual properties of their hybridized identities in an order that signifies the relative importance of the parts. For instance, dance for the camera places dance in a particular relationship to the camera, whereas videodance instates materiality first and dance second. Thus, while the terms are themselves informative, they also constitute specific sites of discourse and practice as defined by their relative order. If this seems overly defined, it is because the theories put forth here are purposefully narrow in scope in order to distance the practice of screendance from other moving image practices about or featuring dance. Focusing on work that is intended to function within a different set of criteria, so as to articulate screendance as a specific practice, I will address here the issue of site-specificity. I stress that in order to rigorously interrogate and theorize the practice of creating technologically mediated or grafted dances, it is important to excavate the relevance of media delivery systems and viewing practices—archives and architectures—for their impact on the reception of moving image work. Further, I explore how meaning is affected by such structures and experiences.

Media of all kinds have historically circulated in deeply coded systems. Cinema, television, newspapers, and the like all are subject to a similar type of scrutiny, one that pre-reads images, both moving and otherwise. We know, for instance, that pictures in newspapers are read in the context of surrounding text, while pictures in a gallery or museum are generally allowed to "speak for themselves." The differences between a thirty-second television commercial and a feature film are obvious, and the images that are contained in each example are necessarily read within the context of their delivery system, including the *architecture* through which they are apprehended.[3]

Perhaps the most critical of all media, language frames the discourse surrounding all art forms, especially in the nascent stages of theoretical evolution. Language describes the materiality and historical affiliations of a movement or practice, either by its specificity or often by omission or unintended usage. In screendance, terminology and semantics have evolved in a way that is perhaps quite accidental, often a case of one community picking up the vernacular usage of a term or phrase and institutionalizing it over the course of a number of iterations, to be adopted by another community of like-minded practitioners.

In Latin America, and Buenos Aires in particular, the term *videodanza* (videodance) is generally applied to all dance made for the screen regardless of the actual method of recording (for instance, video, film, digital media). In this case, the term refers more to a state of mind or a paradigm of production than to the actual materiality or formal qualities of the work in question. The term "dance for camera" is also used in a number of festival situations, although it too has specificity, the implication being that the camera is in service to dance, or is subservient to the dance. Thus, we need to look more deeply at the function of language as it is used to describe the practice of screendance in order to build a foundation for critique and intellectual debate, and to illuminate difference.

I choose to use screendance as a general term because it is the only such term that does not exclude any medium-specific methods of rendering or playback, as long as they are ultimately intended for a screen of some sort.[4] In fact, the term might encompass any form of mediated dance delivered on any kind of screen. This could include animated dance on a computer screen, cine-dance on a projection screen, or videodance projected on a wall or a glass of milk. The term "screen" here is thus loosely applied and open to interpretation: it implies something that is a receptor of an otherwise ephemeral image, and which reifies that image in the process of receiving it. The screen may be an analog device (fabric or wood), or it may be an electronic system (television or computer screen); it may be digital or not. Screendance alludes to the *end point* of a process in which dance is grafted to or merged with techniques of representation particular to viewing on a screen.

General though the parameters of screendance may be, all screens are sites and have specificity and perform those specificities. There is *difference* between the screen of a handheld device and a cinema screen, and those differences conspire to create meaning beyond what is contained within the frame they describe. In the broader discourse of contemporary art, site-specificity is a common condition; it particularly attaches to performative practices but also to postmodern dance, which (as all postmodern practices tend to do) encourages us to look beyond the immediate frame to larger and subsequent frames including site. The site is where the work occurs and forms the architecture against and through which the audience perceives the work. Site provides context. Site-specificity is therefore a way to contextualize a work of art. To apply this to screendance, then, if a dance occurs *only* in the medium of film or video, it must necessarily be critiqued in terms of the architecture of that particular space, even though the tendency is to compare the mediated dance to that of its (often imagined) live version.

Site, as it pertains to screendance, tends to be a moving target. For example, the initial site of production may be an actual physical landscape or architectural space. The next level of mediation (and siting) occurs within the frame of the camera and its particular architecture and material properties. The image is then held or stored for a time in a digital (or filmic) site as it is recorporealized and output to yet another storage medium such as tape or DVD. Finally, it is re-sited *again* at its end point, as a screen image. So, in this sense, the site of screendance is actually a *system* of screendance, built on numerous sites, with the nuances of production and output all contributing to its eventual specificity. These multiple levels and conditions of site-specificity make for a good argument against generalizations about screendance. Site, in screendance, functions as part of an aggregate layering of elements and phenomena, which collectively create both meaning and context. In this case, difference (where it is or is not, how it is or is not) both conveys and disturbs meaning, and sets the parameters for subsequent critique and dialog.

As none of the elements in the construction of a screendance are simply interchangeable without altering meaning or form, each hybrid is doubly specific, and the meaning of each is amplified in that doubling. This means that each viewing situation is also site-specific, and work made initially for the small screen assumes an entirely different set of characteristics when projected in cinematic scale in a festival venue. Of course the opposite is also true: work made for single-channel or festival style screening does not necessarily translate in an installation venue or format without some compromise or alteration. Miwon Kwon proposes that site-specificity in general is undertheorized, and as a result

many artists, critics, historians, and curators, whose practices are engaged in problematizing received notions of site-specificity, have offered alternative formulations, such as context-specific, debate-specific, audience-specific, community-specific, project-based. These terms, which tend to slide into one another at different times, collectively signal an attempt to forge more complex and fluid possibilities for the art-site relationship while simultaneously registering the extent to which the very concept of the site has become destabilized in the past three decades.[5]

Kwon's reading of the field's relationship with site, its shifting ground and need to redefine site as a contingent factor in the production of meaning, is applicable to screendance on numerous levels. The word "screendance," is often used to describe multiple strands of activity, including, first of all, projects made specifically as autonomous works of art, designed especially for the architecture of camera space; and second, work that might be described as *documentary*, which generally follows the traditional approach historically found in documentary filmmaking. Both are featured in festivals dedicated to screendance in the general sense. A third category, *dance documentation*, complicates the discussion because makers of dance documentation often attempt to evolve the material (given the quality and availability of digital cameras and postproduction software) into something more closely resembling a screendance.[6]

There are a number of such works that obscure simple definitions such as "dance for the camera" and "dance documentation." For example, consider the work of Becky Edmunds, based in Brighton in the UK, whose projects powerfully blur the boundaries between documentation, documentary, and screendance. In projects such as *Salt Drawing* (2004), with the choreographer Fiona Wright (described as a documentation by Edmunds), and *El Fuego* (2007), shot in the pampas of Argentina (and which has screened in both "dance on camera" and "videodance" venues), Edmunds resists the architectures of all three conditions—documentation, documentary, and screendance per se—asking the viewer to exercise patience at the lack of customary quick cuts and rapid editing, and creating space to contemplate the nature of her screenic vision. Her works, however, while regularly shown in screendance festivals and which circulate *as* screendance, also, in practice, critique the forms they inhabit.[7]

Despite the porous treatment of boundaries in Edmunds's work, however, screendance tends to be articulated by preset conditions and expectations. For the sake of criticality, it is important to attempt to make some distinctions between areas of research and practice, to define some sites in which the work circulates, and to describe how those sites may contribute to the reading of the work situated therein. There exist under the overarching umbrella of screendance a number of subgenres (see chap. 6), but some

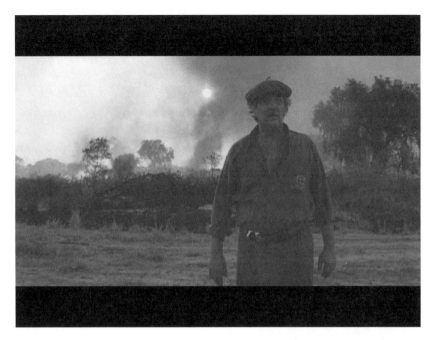

Figure 1.1: *El Fuego* (2007), Video still by Becky Edmunds. Courtesy of the artist.

of these subgenres have other homes as well—such as dance documentation and documentary.[8] Both areas may feature dance and both may have
screens as their end point, yet they are created through processes that are
nonspecific to the art of screendance as a primary site of production. And
although documentation is not the focus of this book, it is valuable to a
discussion of screendance to illuminate some of the more pertinent and/or
salient theories surrounding documentation, its connection to the archive,
and the increasingly porous borders between approaches to inscribing
ephemerality and dancing bodies.

Screendance is a primary site of production—it is an intentional space
with its own architecture and context. It is where the work resides (it is
site-specific). Therefore, all three conditions previously mentioned, documentation, documentary, and screendance per se rely on camera space as
the portal by which dance or bodies in motion are framed. Dance documentation is a functional use of the camera and is of service for two primary
purposes: (1) as a tool by which to circulate a reference of live performance,
choreographic ideas and images in the larger marketplace, and (2) as a tool
to archive and teach choreography in subsequent iterations of live performance. Dance documentation is generally done to preserve a choreography
or performance in its totality and is undertaken during a live performance,

which raises a number of issues. For instance, if a live event is also the material for a simultaneous documentation by one or more recording apparatuses in the theatrical space, then the audience itself is placed in a peculiar position—much like that of the television studio audience. In a sense, they are made particularly aware (by the presence of video cameras) that *this* performance has value beyond its live state and that it is worthy of preservation.

The moving-image documentation of dance has a twofold purpose, one more widely acknowledged than the other. The first is that the performance of the choreography is archived, to be set and reset based on its recorded documentation. What is less recognizable, however, is the way in which the reception of the live performance is altered by the presence of a camera in the theatrical site; how the audience's experience is affected by the presence of and knowledge of contemporaneous recording of a dance event; and how this dialectic affects the audience's perception of the work they are witnessing as it is being recorded. Additionally, dancers are acutely aware of the need for their performance to be "perfect" given the presence of cameras, a phenomenon that exerts considerable external pressure. Such pressure "to perform for the cameras" undoubtedly alters or at least disturbs live performance. An example of this type of recording might circulate beyond its life in the present is the template historically relied upon by broadcast television.

Dance for television is generally shot with multiple cameras placed in strategic locations, including one wide (master) shot. The resulting footage is subsequently edited together in postproduction to give the viewer multiple viewpoints of the dance while still preserving the choreography. Generally, the traditional relationship of the viewer to the stage is maintained. This was the template for the "Dance in America" episodes in PBS's *Great Performances* for many years, as well as other such broadcasts that featured live dance performance edited in real time and taped for future repeated broadcasts. As such, it was similar to the template for sporting events, orchestral performances, or similar situations. In all of these situations, which are predicated on some form of documentation, the end product of the endeavors is contingent on a previously live event and is taken at face value to be an accurate representation of that event. As Sherril Dodds notes in *Dance on Screen* (2001):

> As television has the technological capacity to make a precise reproduction of
> objects and events from the "real world," it is believed to share a close relation-
> ship with reality (Wyver 1986). It is able to construct images that appear to be
> an almost identical copy of the original subject matter. . . . Therefore, on the

surface, it appears that the precise image reproduction of television is more equipped to deal with "re-presenting" reality than dance is.[9]

Television has generally been the benchmark for the archiving of that which is historical. And as such, television documentation has become by default the standard in regard to documenting and preserving dance. Dodds continues:

A fundamental debate for film and television scholars centers on the relation-ship between the image and realty. The complexities of this dialectic are rooted in the ontological questions of whether an objective reality exists, if it can ever be accessed, or whether it will always be mediated by the symbolic structures of language.[10]

I suggest that in the three conditions mentioned earlier, bodies in motion are mediated not only by "the symbolic structures of language" but also by the objectifying architecture of the camera. Thus, documenting and archiving any performed moment predetermines the language by which its qualities will later be further articulated. In other words, the quality of the recording, the placement of the cameras, and the relative success or failure of the performance itself are all framed by the recording of that perfor-mance, regardless of how that moment later circulates as a screenic image.

Since its earliest days, optical media has been used as a method of documentation; recently, digital video has become the preferred technol-ogy. Within the technology of video, the site for storage of the dance becomes the digitally encoded space of the videotape (or as data on a hard drive or other storage device), allowing it to be viewed repeatedly *as it was at the moment of inscription.* The viewing of the dance inscribed in video is always viewed in the present, regardless of the passage of time from its creation. Yet the systems of the moving image are not merely durational; they are also site-specific. For instance, if one considers the theater with its proscenium arch a site for the performance of dance, then one might also consider the camera as a sort of architectural space. Just as the theater has architectural specificity, the same can be said of the camera. The architecture of video, or *video space,* is a construction of transdimen-sionality. Video offers the perception of three-dimensional space in a two-dimensional medium as well as the simultaneous perception of multiple time frames: the viewing present and the past point-of-creation of the original "performance."

The intervention of cameras into a live dance event thereby implies a privileged life beyond the intimate, shared, theatrical experience, and the architecture of replayable media creates the conditions for a reliance on video or digital media as a method of documentation. As a tool, it is not uncommon for choreographers to use video as a feedback device during the choreographic process, and this has been the case since the invention of consumer cameras and portable video recorders. The immediate feedback loop that video provides allows the choreographer to cut and paste ideas, to create a pastiche of phrases, and to use video like an interactive mirror that provides mnemonic markers for movement creation. Thus, the image inscribed on tape serves as an electronic memory of both ideas and execution. Extending this analogy, one might suggest that these electronic or digital markers, because they are imminently retrievable, become privileged in the choreographic process, if only through repetitive viewing.

Repeated viewing of an experience recorded for playback actually embeds in memory that which has been mediated, effectively altering the reception of future live performances. The viewer's experience with mediated images of performance not only inflects the (live) viewing experience but also simultaneously diminishes it, according to Walter Benjamin, who posed a similar problem in his seminal 1936 essay, "The Work of Art in the Age of Mechanical Reproduction." "Even the most perfect reproduction of a work of art is lacking in one element: its presence in time and space, its unique existence at the place where it happens to be." He expands his concerns by stating:

> That which withers in the age of mechanical reproduction is the aura of the work of art. This is a symptomatic process whose significance points beyond the realm of art. One might generalize by saying: the technique of reproduction detaches the reproduced object from the domain of tradition. By making many reproductions it substitutes a plurality of copies for a unique existence.[11]

Benjamin's concern for the welfare of "the original" is exacerbated by documentation. In the digital age, the live event is always in the shadow of mediatization: it is an event in search of an archive.[12]

In dance, there is the tacit assumption that dances performed before a live audience are charged in a way that the same dances played only to a camera are not.[13] This is why videotapes of performances are often accused of (or excused for) being flat and lifeless. If, however, we draw only on traditional theories about dance to understand mediated dance in all its forms, we assume that screendance, lacking liveness, suffers that lack as a kind of loss that occurs in the transition from live to mediated.[14]

Benjamin's concept of the "aura" is important in theorizing the distinctions between live dance, mediated representations of live dance, and screendance, because his theory offers an explanation for the feeling of loss often associated with mediated representations of performance. When we sit in a darkened theater surrounded by others watching the same performance, we are, as a group, experiencing something for the first and only time. The performance may be repeated, but it will never be quite the same. As we disperse after the performance, we take with us individually and collectively the aura of our shared experience, that which bonds us together in that place and time. The aura is what separates a lived experience from one that has been mechanically reproduced, as in videotaped documentation. That unexplainable element that we all know is missing when we view a documentation *of a performance* is the aura. The absence of the aura manifests itself in the form of distance or detachment, the vast and unbearable space between us, the spectator, and the corporeality of the performer.

Benjamin's theory, however, does not address the way in which mediated representations may not simply re-create a live event but rather *recorporealize* it completely. If the relationship between the dance and its mediatized copy is simply documentation, then Benjamin's ideas about the loss of the aura may apply. But dance that is made expressly for the camera—screendance—attempts to *become* the "unique experience" by distancing itself from the original. Indeed, while the original may cease to exist completely as the new work of art is brought into being, the palimpsest of the live dance still lingers beneath its mediatized other. In this case, the live event becomes only a template—source material for the creation of a work in which the architecture of video and the camera are the site to which all elements must conform. If Benjamin's aura attaches at the point of originality, to the original work of art, then certainly we can think of screendance as the original. Given that it is not a copy of a live work nor is it reproducible as a live work, it offers the potential to create intimacy and kinesthetic empathy with its viewer as a primary site of expression. Thus, if the relationship between camera and dance is one intended to produce a mediatized offspring that is singular and not contingent on external means, such as the knowledge of a previous performance, then it is possible that the aura may resurface within the site of screendance.

Dance documentation thus oscillates between the signifier—the mediatized representation of the work—and the thing signified, the original live performance. As much of contemporary culture is experienced via screens, from YouTube to television to iPhones and laptops, the expectation that all performance be available on demand seems to blur the boundaries between the live event and its mediated representation, as if they were one in the same. As live performance tends to fade from memory, documentation is increasingly relied upon as a substitution for the original.

Choreographers rely on it to re-stage work; individuals rely on it as a mnemonic device that aligns graphic images with memories of particular events. And so the signifier in a way becomes the thing itself, increasing in cultural value as the distance between the event and the present increases. Documentation provides cultural proof of the original's existence, archiving the performance or event—dance's equivalent of the museum.[15] This phenomenon also works in the other direction: for instance, the meager documentation of historical dances makes the very ephemerality of dance its most precious commodity—dance's equivalent of a desire predicated on lack. In other words, the scarcity of documentation of early dance works increases the value of what does exist; further, the necessary reliance on still images and anecdotal information makes the work suitably enigmatic.

If documentation has a necessarily contingent relationship to the event, the inverse is also true. Dance artists rely on documentation, using video to re-create choreography and thus circulate their work among potential venues and funding agencies in order to negotiate a subsequent event, which must also be documented so that yet another subsequent event will be possible. On the one hand, documentation performs as both proof of the live occurrence of an event and also as an object of contemplation in which the relative merits of the choreography and performance may be assessed for funding, presenting, and so forth. On the other hand, documentation in lieu of live witnessing is fraught with connotations of insufficiency; it seemingly either elevates or depreciates one's sense of the original, to a certain extent depending on the desire of the viewer. The art historian and critic Amelia Jones writes:

> there is no possibility of an unmediated relationship to any kind of cultural product, including body art. . . . While the live situation may enable the phenomenological relations of flesh-to flesh engagement, the documentary exchange (viewer/reader <—> document) is equally intersubjective. . . . While the viewer of a live performance may seem to have certain advantages in understanding such a context, on a certain level she may find it more difficult to comprehend the histories/narratives/processes she is experiencing until later, when she too can look back and evaluate them with hindsight.[16]

While Jones's commentary is made with a scholar's eye toward theorizing an event, the salient point here is her claim that specific "knowledges" do indeed "develop in relation to the documentary traces of . . . an event." That is, mediated images of performance have a certain value that is separate from but often equally important to live witnessing.

Returning to the circularity of events initiating documentation, the mashing of event/documentation/event continues until what precedes what or what is contingent upon what becomes moot. While the benefits of documentation are clear, what has not been sufficiently interrogated is how the archive itself validates previous events. The critic Rosalind Krauss argues in her essay "Video: The Esthetics of Narcissism":

> [The art world] has become disastrously affected by its relation to mass media. That an artist's work be published, reproduced, and disseminated through the media has become, for the generation that has matured in the course of the last decade, virtually the only means of verifying its existence as art.[17]

Documentation circulates culturally as a kind of artistic capital or collateral, ultimately becoming proof of the artist's existence. As the artist's career progresses, individual events and performances generate a surplus of documentation, often out-massing the original event. Not only does the surplus of documentation continue to expand but so do the possibilities of multipurposing the digital iterations of those documentary traces. This raises questions about the archive itself and its relationship to its iterative event.

In *Archive Fever, A Freudian Impression*, Jacques Derrida traces the term "archive" to its Greek origins, where it meant "a house, a domicile, an address, the residence of the superior magistrates, the *archons*, those who commanded."[18] The residents of these domiciles, due to their political power, were entrusted with official documents to be kept in the place that was their home: "Entrusted to such archons, these documents in effect speak the law . . . they needed at once a guardian and a localization. . . . The dwelling, the place where they dwell permanently, marks this institutional passage from private to public."[19] Permanence, in a digital culture, is a moving target; the bricks and mortar dwellings, the archives that Derrida describes, all are increasingly giving way to online or digital venues. As more and more archives become open source, the passage from private to public becomes less local, less site-specific. The archive that is accessible via the Internet is no longer geographically bound but global in its reach. To a certain extent, the digitization and decentralization of the archive further obscures the question of what is archivable.

Derrida goes on to quote Freud, from *Civilization and its Discontents*: "'In none of my previous writings have I had so strong a feeling as now that what I am describing is common knowledge and that I am using up paper and ink and, in due course, the compositor's and printer's work and material in order to expound things which are, in fact, self-evident.'"[20] On one hand, Freud is worried that he is wasting resources in archiving his writings. On the other hand, he is seemingly hedging his bet, the rationale being that if his research turns out to be an "original proposition," then the investment will prove to be wise.

In a sense, this is the dichotomy that we have engaged as artists in the twenty-first century. What do we archive, how do we archive? Derrida states:

> archival technology no longer determines, will never have determined, merely the moment of the conservational recording, but rather the very institution of the archivable event. It conditions not only the form, or the structure that prints, but the printed content of the printing . . . what is no longer archived in the same way is no longer lived in the same way. . . . Because everything is archived, everything is archivable. The gap between art and life as mediated by technology diminishes and experience is reduced to retrievable bit of data.[21]

"Archive fever" displaces experience and privileges playback over liveness, or as Derrida warns, "incites forgetfulness, amnesia, [and] the annihilation of memory."[22] So as documentation becomes more and more pervasive, it becomes less clear whether the event inspires the documentation or the possibility of documentation inspires the event.

While employing similar tools as documentation, screendance occupies a wholly different architecture: though still ultimately contributing a kind of archive, screendance distances itself from the documentation of live theatrical dance by both intent and by deploying technologies of representation. If documentation is subsequent to the moment of performance, then screendance is preceded by the moment of performance. In its ideal state, screendance is not reproducible as a live work; such is the gestalt of movement, media, and editing. Instead, it is a hybrid contextualized by the medium and method of recording, and as such exists *only* in its mediated form. It is not a substitute for, or in conflict with, the live theatrical performance of a dance but rather a wholly separate and equally viable way of creating art works. Screendance, sometimes referred to as "dance for the camera," may be better described as *dance by the camera*. That is, while the intent of the dancer or choreographer may be to situate the movement within the frame of the camera, it is ultimately the frame that defines the boundaries and reproducibility of the movement. Screendance, then, relies on the specific ability of media to recompose, re-edit, and ultimately re-create a dancing body in a way that distances itself from the historical realism of documentation and the desire to faithfully and accurately archive the integrity of both choreography and performance in a live setting.

Even though the dance may be made *for* the camera (intent), it is ultimately made *by* the camera (reification) as it scans the body, articulating both presence and absence via the recorded image. In this case, the site of production is literally media space.

Media space (or video space) is a complex site that has been mapped and remapped since media technologies first became available.[23] However, the site of media is one in which the production of the media object and the reception of that object must be considered as part of the *media process*. Just as writing produces books, which are different than magazines or comic strips, composition for a screen produces viewable objects with specificity and difference as well. The reception and viewing of those objects may either reinforce or distort the original intent of the work in the same way as reading a poem on a roadside billboard originally intended for the intimacy of a chapbook will skew the experience of those lines. Cinema was the end point for the dances of Gene Kelly, Fred Astaire, and Busby Berkeley, and had its own architectural viewing space. Movies of the type and era in which Kelly and others labored were historically viewed in the dark, surrounded by a number of other viewers. This larger-than-life experience of moviegoing contributed greatly to a sense of both spectacle and community. Changes in technology, however, have created multiple viewing paradigms through which viewers may adapt their viewing strategies, and these strategies have infiltrated all levels of media viewing, including screendance.

For example, screendance festivals generally follow the historical model of cinema, projecting work on a large screen for multiple viewers simultaneously. By contrast, the films one may encounter in the institutionalized setting of the festival may also be viewed outside of that setting on a television, computer screen, or handheld device. In regard to scale and a sense of community, this is a comparatively intimate experience. There are other characteristics particular to both models that differentiate the experiences and attach them to other historical modes. The festival screening attaches to issues of curation, institutionalization, and competition, while the model in which one might view work streaming on the Internet or via a DVD aligns itself with the utopian idealism of early video art practice—a kind of media egalitarianism that functions outside of the traditional producer/receiver paradigm. Screendance flows easily between both models of circulation and distribution. Thus, although these phenomena would suggest that both the viewing and reception of screendance is similar to other practices (such as Hollywood film production and distribution) in the digital age, there are considerable material and esthetic considerations that mark screendance as a specific site of inscription, production, and distribution in its relationship to archives and architecture alike, especially when it progresses from concerns particular to issues of liveness.

The nature of live dance is that each performance of a work has a unique life of its own, a dangerous, flexible life. Live dance exists with the understanding that no two performances are ever the same, that the threat of failure is imminent: failure to remember, failure to perform, failure to arrive onstage at the specified location as per the choreography. The phenomenon is exceedingly apparent, for instance, when the dancer in a role changes for any reason. The dance and the choreography are together a living, organic being. The mediatized performance, or the one committed to media, inscribed electronically, digitally, or otherwise, is a permanent record, and even though subject to deterioration in a number of ways, it is fundamentally fixed, no longer subject to the vagaries of the body, space, or time. Both documentation and screendance offer permanency; they are as fixed as media can be. While, as Benjamin proposes, live events archived on film somehow diminish the original, screendance *is* the original and therefore cannot diminish itself. To use Baudrillard's description of the "hyperreal" as a guide, the creation of a screendance does not efface a live version in favor of a mediatized version; it effaces *itself* in the creation of the truer than true, the performance of a body that cannot and does not exist.[24] While the movement encountered in a screendance may be performed by real bodies in real time and space, it is done solely to provide material for the screendance. The screendance is predicated on the erasure of live performance's notions of linearity and temporality, as well as the fracturing of choreographic unity, for a new and different unity specific to the architecture and archival concerns of media space. What we see in viewing the finished work/screendance is simultaneously a documentation of a performed moment and also a record of the subsequent recorporealization and editing decisions made in the process of creating the screendance. Performance attaches to both the moment of creation—the initial rendering of the movement via the camera—and also to the extended process of reconstruction that is manifest as the finished screendance. The subsequent act of viewing a screendance requires the viewer (audience) to reimagine the materiality of dance as well as the specificity of dance in its mediated form. Matthew Reason and Dee Reynolds propose that

> We might comfortably recognize that audiences adopt different viewing strategies for different arts forms or different platforms (cinema, broadcast television, recorded media, reality television, live theatre or dance performance) in a manner that is suggestive of a virtuosity in audiencing. What the collective debate about screen dance audiences might also indicate is that as art practices

increasingly operate slippages across forms so audiences become attuned to an ambiguity of form and adopt a hybridity of viewing strategies.[25]

The authors point out that the way in which audiences encounter screendance requires considerable flexibility, though not all cues are readily readable by all audiences, and not all audiences are immediately flexible without some additional contextualization on the part of the presenting institution. Making meaning from screendance relies on a number of signals and cues that come not only from the work but from the architecture of the viewing space and a number of other phenomena that occur as screendance gestures toward its public.

Screendance opens its subject up to analysis and interaction from multiple points of view, not only in terms of physical locations but metaphorical ones as well. Cinematic points of view may encompass poetic or abstract representations of place as well as make visual reference to an emotional state of being. Conversely, live dance unfolds in real, linear time and is intended to be consumed in a similar manner. It is constructed as an accretion of interlocking pieces, built in analog fashion, as if brick upon brick. The dance made for the architecture of the camera, however, is made of individual choreographic events that exist in parallel: not intersecting, not necessarily accruing meaning, context or linearity until recomposed in the editing process. The cinematic experience, beginning with the camera's framing of its subject, allows for a constantly shifting, ever-fluid definition of place and time.

Cameras, as an integral component of media space, are both telescopic and microscopic in their ability to extend vision and facilitate a kind of seeing that is a manifestation of our desire to draw phenomena closer to us.[26] This attempt to create intimacy is destabilized in the translation or migration to movement in media space. The prosthetic capability of cameras and lenses nevertheless presents seductive possibilities for a particular *kind* of intimacy. In the Renaissance, artists relied on optical devices that included lenses, such as the camera obscura, to assist in articulating and re-creating the natural world.[27] Optical devices, however, can focus or defocus the natural world, rendering it more or less accurately. And in the case of screendance, editing and postproduction create the potential for distancing the mediated image from its original source, thereby effectively extending the body's natural abilities.

For example, *Leap Into the Void* (1960), by the French artist Yves Klein (1928–62), is a highly realistic visual image, made possible by photo montage processes that predated Photoshop. It offers a compelling visual metaphor in which we are left to wonder about Klein's inevitable landing, one

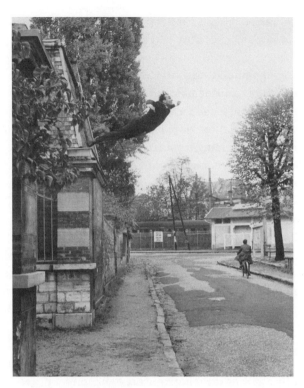

Figure 1.2: Leap into the Void (1960) Yves Klein, photograph by Harry Shunk (1924–2006)

Image copyright © The Metropolitan Museum of Art/Art Resource, NY Klein, Yves (1928–1962) © ARS, NY. Harry Shunk (1924–2006) ©, and John Kender (1937–c.1983) ©. Leap into the Void. 1960.

Gelatin silver print. 25.9 x 20.0 cm (10 3/16 x 7 7/8 in.). Purchase, The Horace W. Goldsmith Foundation Gift, through Joyce and Robert Menschel, 1992 (1992.5112) May have restrictions.

Image copyright © The Metropolitan Museum of Art/Art Resource, NY The Metropolitan Museum of Art, New York, NY, U.S.A.

© 2010 Artists Rights Society (ARS), New York/ADAGP, Paris

that never comes.[28] Klein's piece shows us that cameras serve to render movement (for instance) either as it is or as it might be. These prosthetic devices, created to assist in facilitating a realistic view of the world, may be also used to inscribe images of movement that are at odds with or abstracted from the natural or realistic world. In screendance, we can identify a broad spectrum of approaches to such challenges, from realist to abstract and hybrids thereof.

The choreographer Merce Cunningham, who worked extensively in the field of screendance, often explored the difference between the site of the theater and the site of the screen, as in his 1979 work *Locale* with director

Charles Atlas. The title of the piece refers to the fact that it is not a work for the theater, rather that the dance exists entirely within the purview or *locale* of the camera. The camera allowed Cunningham and Atlas to explore time, space, energy, and movement in ways that traditional theatrical space completely disallowed. The dance writer David Vaughan states: "In the previous pieces, Cunningham and Atlas had dealt principally with movement within the frame rather than movement of the frame—using that is to say, a mostly stationary camera with no fancy editing. Now they were ready to explore the possibilities of a moving camera."[29] In *Locale,* the camera moves through the space at breakneck speed as dancers randomly appear and disappear from the frame. The effect is quite the opposite of the entrances and exits one expects in the theater. It feels as if the camera is in a sense "discovering" the movement already in progress. Vaughan states that Cunningham had an "instinctive understanding" that the language of video was quite different than that of the stage, "realizing for instance, that time can be treated elliptically because the spectator absorbs informa-tion much faster than in the theater, and that space appears to widen out from the small aperture of the screen, giving an illusion of greater depth than in fact exists."[30] As Cunningham and his collaborators realized, media space as a site for choreography is a malleable space for the exploration of dance as subject, object, and metaphor. The practice of articulating this site is one in which the very nature of choreography and the action of dance may be questioned, deconstructed, and *re*-presented as an entirely new hybrid form through experimentation with camera angles, shot composition, location and postproduction techniques.

As the quality and resolution of video has improved in recent years and digital technology has infiltrated film, the boundaries between film and video practice have begun to diminish. Still, each has its own specificity, history, and formal qualities. Screendance, when sited within the milieu of digital technologies, places itself in the discourse of contemporary media practice and therefore in the discourse of popular culture and media theory as well. It also anchors itself in the history of video art and its self-imposed distance from film history. Film has its own particular historical narrative and technologies of representation, as does video. Video practice is distinct from that of film, both materially and historically (see chap. 4). In the earli-est days of video art, this distancing was a strategy purposefully employed by video artists. And, as Marshal McLuhan proposed in 1964, the medium *was* the message:

> In a culture like ours, long accustomed to splitting and dividing all things as
> a means of control, it is sometimes a bit of a shock to be reminded that, in

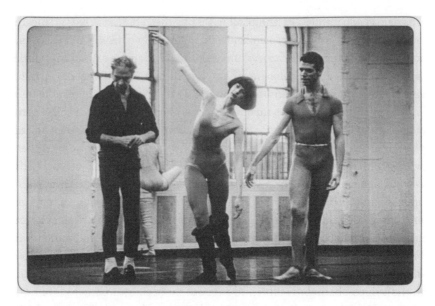

Figure 1.3: *Locale* rehearsal with Merce Cunningham (1979), photograph by Art Becofsky, courtesy of the artist.

operational and practical fact, the medium is the message. This is merely to say that the personal and social consequences of any medium—that is, of any extension of ourselves—result from the new scale that is introduced into our affairs by each extension of ourselves, or by any new technology.[31]

If the "extension of ourselves" that McLuhan describes is taken at face value, we must also consider intent and context as a part of the equation. That said, the medium that produces the message that McLuhan suggests, extends even beyond the technologies of representation to the conceptual foundation of works of art. It also extends then to the means and method of circulation of a given work of art. In articulating a theory of screendance, the medium remains a defining characteristic of the message.

CHAPTER 2
Mediated Bodies

From Photography to Cine-Dance

Over the years, as cinema and dance have traversed modernism, they have engaged in an almost unbroken courtship, each gazing at the other and ultimately appropriating both technique and style from the object of their affection.[1] Indeed, there have been significant moments in the histories of dance and the optical mediums—such as cinema—when the two co-mingled their methodologies, resulting in profound effects in each field. For example, prior to the birth of cinema, the photographer Eadweard Muybridge turned his attentions to dancers and other bodies to articulate his ideas about sequential inscription of motion. As cinema emerged, Thomas Edison and others, including Georges Méliès and the Lumières in France, began looking toward dance as they created the first moving pictures that marked the passing of time through bodies in motion. Later, the silent films of Chaplin, Buster Keaton, Harold Lloyd, and others were a fertile field for early hybridity in which movement and cinema each articulated the other's potential. Movement was literally used to advance the narrative as well as the passage of time within the films, while cinema provided the site in which actors could explore the specificity of the frame, as separate and different from the live space of theater. Finally, as dance moved into the contemporary or modern era, live theatrical dance mimicked cinematic editing styles. Later, live dance mimicked the French New Wave-inspired jump-cut by using lighting techniques, which allowed shifts in fields of activity to occur in darkness and reemerge in light, thereby mirroring the nonlinear propensity of film and/or video editing and remediating it for the stage.

The histories of dance have exerted a particular influence on the way in which the histories of screendance have been inscribed. Screendance has been typically historicized as a subgenre of dance history. Two books in particular come to mind in that regard: the first, Judy Mitoma's *Envisioning Dance on Film and Video*, clearly states its purpose in the title: to articulate a narrative in which "dance" appears on screen in any and all genres and conditions.[2] The second, *Dance on Screen*, by Sherril Dodds, features an equally performative title and further states its narrative desire in the first chapter's subhead: "Histories of Dance on Screen."[3] These two examples are representative of the field's reliance on or desire to inscribe a historical narrative dependent on "dance" as the motivating and/or decisive factor in a binary model. In other words, it is a kind of archeological undertaking in which all media sources are examined for the presence of dance and subsequently cataloged or indexed under the broadest of terms such as "dance on camera." Such indexes most often function in a strictly historical framework. In Virginia Brooks's chapter "From *Méliès* to Streaming Video: A Century of Moving Dance Images" from Mitoma's *Envisioning Dance*, Brooks meticulously tells the story of how and when various dances were recorded for playback but makes no substantive points about difference, either material or otherwise, instead simply stating the facts as they relate to the archeology of her research. Earlier in the book, Brooks offers an actual timeline ("A Century of Dance and Media") that lays out *"landmark dance films/videos"* and *"advances in film/video technology"* but does not make any claim as to what constitutes the status of "landmark" in relation to dance film and video practice. This attempt to organize a history and articulate important contributions is most often undertaken without any accompanying theoretical foundation and is largely predicated on matters of taste.[4]

In gathering examples with which to populate a history of "dance on camera," Brooks exemplifies how the net has been cast very wide, with virtually any and all film/dance/moving image combinations cited as part of the nascent canon regardless of genre, style, intent, or contextualization outside of dance's own closed historical narrative. While indexes of dance on film and/or video are useful to an extent, they are still an arbitrary designation that offers little in the way of information about form, content, meaning, and most important, context, and do little to engage intertextual and/or interhistorical narratives from the theories and histories of film, the visual arts, and other synergistic practices.

A common perception of the historical continuum of dance on screen places the genesis of the form in the mid-twentieth century, with Busby Berkeley's Hollywood musicals forming the pivot point of one strand of activity, and Maya Deren's experimentalist films its counterpoint.[5] Although this assumption articulates a particular dialectic regarding style, it is far too simplistic to serve as the entire narrative of the trajectory of screendance. The Berkeley/Deren pairing is convenient for many reasons, as it is predicated not just on a specific definition of "choreography" but also on the idea that choreography and film began a courtship in the era of Hollywood musicals that emblematized the potential for the symbiotic relationship of dance and film. In this view, "choreography" must be fore-grounded in order for a work to be considered *as* screendance and that the presence of dancing bodies with or without agency, either as part of a narrative arc or simply for dance's poetic visual impact, is sufficient to contextualize a work as screendance.

The pairing of films by Busby Berkeley and Maya Deren as oppositional forces (Hollywood vs. avant-garde) is certainly instructive in fashioning a history and/or theory of screendance, yet this pairing does not represent a genesis point nor does it offer much in the way of illumination. In fact, Berkeley and Deren are late entries along the continuum of production that flows from a rhizomatic network of sources; the relationship of dance and the architectural specificity of the camera begins far earlier than the work of either director, with a different set of desires, intentions, and purposes.[6] Both Berkeley and Deren were concerned with using dance to further a narrative or to emulate or extend preexisting structures, but the work that preceded these genres—Muybridge, Edison, and others—was less con-cerned with narrative arc than with the phenomenology of bodies in motion as apprehended by optical technologies. These moments of realization, in which the camera acted as a prosthetic that extended the viewer's ability to perceive movement, require us to rethink the historiographies of dance and its relationship to media, as well as the histories of the moving image. The experimental works of Muybridge and Edison prefigure a burgeoning desire to apprehend and frame movement that characterizes a predomi-nance of modernist artistic endeavors in the twentieth century.

Since the earliest days of photography, artists working with optical mediums have been fascinated by the possibility of recording human move-ment, in particular, that of dance. Early photographs of Isadora Duncan and Loïe Fuller attest to the immediate rapport between camera and dancer, an extension perhaps of the historic desire on the part of painters and sculptors, both prior to and after the birth of photography, to represent dance through their own methods of reproduction. The index of early photographic images of dancers such as Duncan and Fuller further verifies dance's willing and often eager submission of itself to mediation, first in still form and later as moving image. It is apparent in many such early photos that the dancer is not simply posing for the camera but rather *dancing* for the camera. The photographer, composing the frame, actively

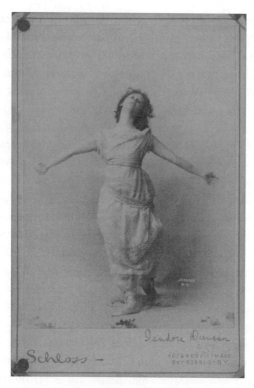

Figure 2.1: Untitled photograph of Isadora Duncan (1898), photograph by A. Schloss, courtesy Jerome Robbins Dance Division, The New York Public Library for the Performing Arts, Astor, Lenox and Tilden Foundations

participates in the "choreography" of the picture. The resulting image is a moment of choreography, suspended in time much like a single frame of film lifted out of succession.

Eadweard Muybridge was an English photographer whose work documenting animal and human motion anticipated cinema as well as the cinematic fascination with movement. He invented a timing mechanism that allowed numerous cameras to make photographs in rapid succession, capturing human and animal locomotion in a way never before possible. In presenting movement in chronological photographic frames, he was able to simultaneously reference the subject's past, present, and future in a single image set.

Muybridge chose to use both dancers and non-dancers in his motion studies; he was not concerned with choreography per se but with the camera's ability to articulate difference between frames of movement. This phenomenon—the visualization of the passage of time via the objectification of movement—occurred during a period when few people had

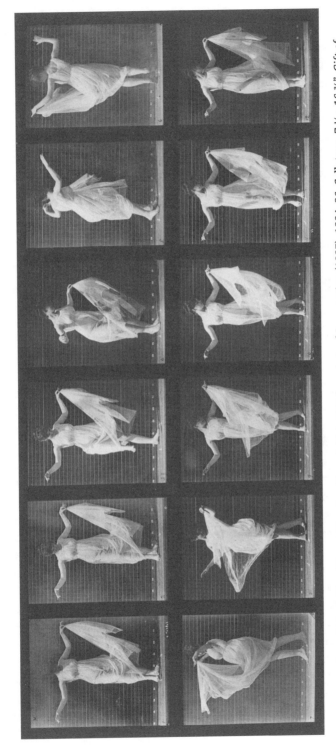

Figure 2.2: Eadweard Muybridge, Woman Dancing (Fancy): Plate 187 from Animal Locomotion (1887). 1884–86. Collotype, 7 ¼ x 16 ¾". Gift of Mrs. Jane K. Murray, The Museum of Modern Art, NY, U.S.A. Digital Image c. The Museum of Modern Art/Licensed by SCALA/Art Resource, NY

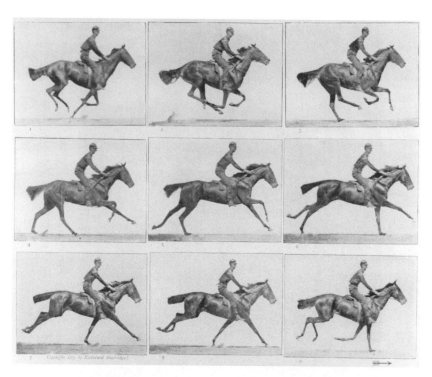

Figure 2.3: Eadweard Muybridge Transverse-Gallop, photograph, 1887. From "Animals in Motion." Photo Credit: Image Select/Art Resource.

experienced in three-dimensional reality what Muybridge's pictures were able to extrapolate in two dimensions. For example, it was not until 1869 that the first transcontinental railroad was completed, wherein the traveler could feel the novel experience of past, present, and future collapsing upon one another while remaining seated, relatively motionless, a passenger on a train, which moved through space and time faster than heretofore imagined.[7] And it was not until the early 1900s that the art world began to address the phenomena of movement in a two-dimensional picture plane via Cubism, in which the artist depicts the subject from a multitude of viewpoints, thus mimicking, to a certain extent, the phenomena for which Muybridge helped to lay the foundation.

Muybridge published eleven volumes of photographic studies called *Animal Locomotion: An Electro-photographic Investigation of Consecutive Phases of Animal Movements, 1872–1885*; yet, while Muybridge often worked with animals, many of his subjects were athletes and people performing simple, pedestrian movements for the camera.[8] In 1879 he invented the zoöpraxiscope, a device that allowed figures in motion to be projected on a screen and which directly foreshadowed motion pictures. His work thus initiated the transition from still photography toward the narrative, sequential structure of film.

In the same era, Thomas Edison, experimenting with recording successive images via a single camera, developed his Kinetoscope. Edison was fascinated with inscribing motion with his new invention and remarked in 1888: "I am experimenting upon an instrument which does for the eye what the phonograph does for the ear, which is the recording and reproduction of things in motion."[9] In that same year, Muybridge met with Edison to pitch his idea for a collaboration between Muybridge's zoöpraxiscope and Edison's phonograph, but this partnership never materialized. As early as 1894, Edison began making silent films featuring dance at his Black Maria Film Studio and soon embarked upon his own experiments with film and sound, many of which took dancers as their subject.[10] Because Edison's still-young technology required that the camera be anchored to a tripod, it was the dancer who supplied motion to the frame, thereby amplifying the camera's ability to comprehend movement ⬤.

Although these projects could be considered as seminal cine-dance works, it is important to note that Edison's films were illustrative of a working theory and not created as works of art. Similarly, Muybridge's sequential studies of bodies in motion were not created as autonomous art photography but rather in the service of science (although they garnered much attention from subsequent artists and choreographers). Nevertheless, Muybridge's motion studies have become, over the years, recontextualized *as* art objects, and they figure significantly in theory related to the intersection of dance and technology.[11]

Audiences also encountered one of the first demonstrations of Edison's Kinetoscope in 1894, which featured a short film of a music hall performer, Annabelle Moore, re-creating one of her stage dances. Moore's work follows the style of Loïe Fuller, employing sweeping arm motions to move the diaphanous folds of her costume in swirling, flowing arcs. The piece begins with a fixed shot of Annabelle, who is already in motion. The stationary camera frames the dancer head to toe throughout the duration of the film while the dancer moves around a central axis, her voluptuous costume occasionally filling the screen. Edison subsequently hand-colored the film to mimic the light projections, made famous by Fuller and her many imitators, that cast changing colors of light onto the dancer's costume. The film ends abruptly, cutting her off mid-movement ⬤.

Edison, like Muybridge, was not interested in dance per se, but bodies in motion helped to demonstrate the qualities to which his early experiments in motion pictures aspired: the depiction of movement in real time and the cinematic exploration of the human condition. Some of Edison's other early film experiments form a virtual archive of fin de siècle world dance, featuring Japanese dancers, Hopi and Sioux Indians, and perhaps the first filmed male duet, an 1895 film (listed in the Library of Congress only as "Dickson experimental sound film") in which two men dance cheek to cheek while a violinist plays in the background ●.

Meanwhile, other artists clearly aligned with artistic production used similar vision-enhancing technologies to other ends. The painter Thomas Eakins collaborated with Muybridge in the 1880s and went on to develop his own camera, which allowed him to record multiple, sequential images in the same photograph. Eakins used photography the way that Renaissance painters used lenses—to extend the possibilities of vision—though photography was a catalyst for his paintings, a way to capture the hidden truths of movement invisible to the naked eye. His photographic studies of bodies in motion, often made for the sole purpose of migrating those images to the canvas, are in retrospect contextualized as art in discussions of the history of photography. It is in these moments of overlap (particularly in the work of Eakins) that the monolithic practices of painting, dancing, and the nascent art of photography begin to blend into a practice that is both pluralistic and overlooked for its significance to the history of screendance. And it is in moments of overlap that we find a synergistic and nonhierarchical relationship between the depiction of bodies in motion and the method of recording and inscribing those actions. In other words, they are not coded as dance film or dance photography, nor are they narrative or simply documentary; they exist instead in the spaces in between, as liminal artifacts of collisions between disparate mediums that result in real hybrids of form and content.

Both Muybridge's and Edison's work (as well as that of the Lumières', Étienne-Jules Marey, Thomas Eakins, and other early adopters and inventors of cinematic or photographic technologies) created a purely conceptual paradigm for the investigation of the human form in motion, with no reliance on narrative or any other constructions associated with the movement of bodies in other mediums such as literature, drama, dance, or cinema. As is often the case in the early stages of technological development, the image or object produced via an inchoate technology was secondary to scientific innovation and quantification. It was not until later, as the optical arts developed, that filmmakers fluent in cinema and photography began to create works of art with the new technologies. That fluency, coupled with intentionality, produced artworks in which technology became the means to an artistic, esthetic end.

Roland Barthes, in *Camera Lucida, Reflections on Photography*, points out that "at first photographic implements were related to . . . the machinery of precision: cameras . . . were clocks for seeing."[12] This conflation of photography with the precision of timekeeping is quite informative in regard to the inscription of dancing bodies on film. Dancing bodies are, in fact, a kind of timekeeping device. Perhaps a better metaphor might be to say that dancing bodies, in relation to the moving image, are keepers of the metronomic *passage* of time. Bodies in motion *prove* the thesis of motion picture technologies as they virtually illustrate the movement of linear time. The visualization of choreography on film reinforces that what we are a witness to is indeed the *passing* of time. This sort of concrete use of dance as a metronome to prove cinema is the earliest incarnation of the relationship of dance to the moving image, but kept in context, it is still closer to science than to art ❾.

From the turn-of-the-century work of Georges Méliès, the French filmmaker, and the American D. W. Griffith, dance continued to be featured prominently in motion pictures in the early twentieth century, a partnership often thought to culminate in the Hollywood musicals and the Busby Berkeley spectacles of the 1930s. Yet dance has never been far from the surface of cinematic exploration. In Griffith's *Intolerance*, made in 1916 and featuring the Ruth St. Denis Dancers (who were also among the earliest performers for Edison's Kinetoscope), dance becomes a recurring motif, contributing to the film's status as one of the earliest examples of a *hybrid cinema*, nonlinear and metaphoric, utilizing cross-cutting in a way that precedes the technique in common practice by decades.[13] Méliès also prominently features dance in his 1903 film, *The Magic Lantern*, as well as in a number of others. Méliès, who had a strong interest in the ballets of Paris, utilized movement in his work to disrupt and reconfigure both time and space. He moved freely between working in the theater and film, and each informed the other in their approach to spectacle.[14] Additionally, the films of Méliès and Griffith employ techniques of pastiche and appropriation that would come to be recognizable postmodern tendencies. Their intertextual linking of the live and the mediatized resonates with the contemporary practice of screendance, and this is an example of the roots of screendance and of the courtship of dance by photographic representation present at the birth of cinema.

The occasional attempt to craft a timeline of screendance practice by artists and critics usually places Méliès, Edison, and others, including Norman McLaren, in a narrative that subsequently jumps abruptly to Maya Deren's *A Study in Choreography for Camera* as the pivotal work of dance on film, the film that comes closest to a genesis point for contemporary screendance.

This tendency leaves a large gap in the historical continuum, though more in the historiography than in the history itself. Deren's work is an evolution not only of her own understanding of early film and dance cultures but also of her proximity to and inheritance from other artists working within similar milieus.

Indeed, there is a bridge between Thomas Edison's fin-de-siècle cinematic movement portraits and Deren's *A Study in Choreography for Camera*, one that that has been often overlooked for its significance to screendance. While this bridge is inhabited by Méliès, Griffith, and other early auteurs of cinema, there is still more connective tissue in the silent films of cinematic performers such as Charlie Chaplin and Buster Keaton. The Chaplin and Keaton films are predicated on a particular type of physicality and an acknowledgement of cinema's ability to create and illuminate movement through editing. This is work made for the camera in the same way that later so-called dance films were created without a prior life on the stage. However, this bridge between cinema's earliest architects and Maya Deren and others is also populated by another group of artists who have been equally absent from the screendance narrative. That said, it was a bridge crowded with *visual artists* as well, including Marcel Duchamp, Fernand Léger, and Man Ray, most of whom have been elided or minimized in accounts of the development of screendance.

While Deren certainly created a stylistic breakthrough in her work with the choreographer and dancer Talley Beatty, her approach to filmmaking was built on a foundation of cinematic visuality put in place by her predecessors. Deren's first and best-known film, *Meshes of the Afternoon* (1943), was aligned with the American avant-garde film movement; yet there are echoes of European avant-garde cinema in her films as well, especially from the likes of Léger (*Ballet Mechanique*, 1924), Buñuel, and Dali (*Un Chien Andalou*, 1928). While these artists—who contributed to both the language of cinema as well as to the development of Deren's esthetic— made films, it is important to note that they were not filmmakers as such. They were artists trained in other practices who brought an outsider esthetic to filmmaking. This theme of artists from other media moving with great fluidity into and out of media-based practices recurs throughout the history of experimental film and video art as well as the current practice of screendance. It contributes to a kind of mongrelism within film and video practice that often pushes back against the purity of those forms of expression and adds to the development of screen esthetics, all the while reifying a porous, permeable boundary between the visual arts and the moving image. Even though this kind of cross-pollination of art to film and video (and vice versa) has been acknowledged by the histories of both genres, screendance and dance in general have been perhaps less gracious in their acknowledgement of the impact of the fine arts on their respective visualities.

Again, Maya Deren's work did not spring from a vacuum, fully formed as the prescient image of cine-dance to come nor is it aligned solely with the histories and practices of the nascent modern dance of the mid-century. Instead, it rose to its elevated status from a milieu of cinematic experimentation in which surrealism, painting, and the performative screen presences of Chaplin, Keaton, and others co-mingled with a fin de siècle fascination with movement exemplified by the Futurists and Cubists. In *Envisioning Dance on Film and Video*, Amy Greenfield notes, "[Buster] Keaton was a major inspiration for artists when Deren made *A Study*."[15] She also cites the "trick film" innovations of Keaton, specifically cutting from one location to another in a dislocation of site, while maintaining continuity of movement. This technique is particularly evident in *The Cook* (1918), Keaton's film collaboration with Roscoe (Fatty) Arbuckle. Here, Keaton, playing the waiter, begins an improvisation with a dancing girl in the restaurant and continues as a solo by Keaton in the kitchen—without losing the continuity of the movement. The dance then becomes a duet with Arbuckle, but is seen in separate frames and punctuated by Arbuckle's tossing of food-laden plates across frames to Keaton (again cutting on movement that seamlessly continues from frame to frame).

While critics and theorists including Greenfield and Virginia Brooks have described the points of tangency between Deren and other early filmmakers, the foundation of visuality laid by artists like Keaton and Chaplin has not been thoroughly illustrated for its impact on subsequent "dance" films. That sense of visual space is one in which linearity and cinematic narrative play a game of hide-and-seek with the viewer. One moment it is in evidence; the next it is pitched in favor of surreal interludes entirely lacking in the logic that both precedes and follows it. These are the same sorts of digressive interludes that interrupt and disturb the flow of modernism itself, and ultimately lead to postmodernism and other practices associated with the lingua franca of the visual arts that are farther down the path of screendance. These digressive moments, such as the dancing dinner rolls scene in Charlie Chaplin's silent film, *The Gold Rush* (1925) ⬎, exemplify a kind of fragmentation at odds with the traditions of storytelling in real, linear time that was the common method of the era. In *The Gold Rush*, Chaplin's Tramp is stranded in a remote cabin in the Yukon; there he encounters a number of unlikely situations that result in vignettes framing his comic physicality. Although *The Gold Rush* is a narrative film, it is full of poetic and digressive incursions, perhaps the most well known and pertinent of which is the "Oceana Rolls" scene. Chaplin performs a tabletop dance sequence in which he anthropomorphizes a matching set of dinner rolls stuck on the ends of two forks. The scene begins with a wide shot of his three guests and himself at a fully laden table. As Chaplin moves a candlestick and other objects out of the way, the scene cuts to a close-up: we see that Chaplin has created a sort of shadow box or puppet space by using his torso as the theatrical space (or backdrop) for the dancing rolls. The quality of the movement encompasses both the manipulation of the fork/ rolls as legs and also Chaplin's bobbing head and torso, which ultimately are read in conjunction with the dancing appendages he has created. What we see is a kind of hybrid body, made possible by Chaplin's virtuosic performance and by the cameras framing of the scene. The scene is shot in one long take, and there are no cuts between the start of the close-up and the bow at the end of the "dance." Subsequent to this digressive performance, the film picks up the narrative where it left off, making no notice of what has just occurred.

Formally, this strategy is played out in contemporary screendance works, and although *The Gold Rush* has never been situated in the discourse of screendance as such, I intend to appropriate this scene and the larger film of which it is a part in order to illuminate a thread that connects such modernist cinematic constructions with the way in which screendance historically has inserted dance into unlikely scenarios and to claim this scene as a part of screendance history and vernacular. We can look at Chaplin's work *as if* it is screendance only if we have first created a context by which to do so. In other words, we can appropriate and decontextualize the clip because we are recontextualizing it within a frame of reference that supports our theory.

The narrative in Chaplin's film helps viewers to situate themselves as sympathetic to the character. Nonetheless, Chaplin's "cinematic body" disrupts the viewer's sense of self through his embodiment of a particular sort of kinesthetic performance. The film historian Tom Gunning argues that Chaplin's work presents us with something new on screen, "the body of modernity." Chaplin's cinematic performance in film after film exemplifies a "balletic-acrobatic-mechanical physical process [which] seem[s] to remain divorced from achieving anything," roughly the equivalent of the interminable sense of futility found in Samuel Beckett's work for stage, a metaphysical musing of screenic corporeality. Gunning states that "Chaplin was the first performer . . . who transferred the mechanical rhythm inherent in the cinema machine, both camera and projector, into a performance style for film." Chaplin is a pivotal figure for any new theory of screendance, as his performance is inextricably linked to the materiality of its inscription. Gunning continues:

> Chaplin's cinematic body defies verbal description—and that's the point. His body transforms before our eyes . . . Chaplin's physical nature also exceeds his human identity and transforms itself into the mechanical . . . and] seems at points to disaggregate itself, with limbs operating independently of each other, or to merge with other bodies and create new creatures. Chaplin slides up and down the great chain of being, achieving a plastic ontology in which inanimate objects become bodily appendages, and the body itself suddenly seems inert . . . Chaplin's art does not consist simply in a new physical language that speaks to modern experience, or in a power to imitate and redefine the rhythms of that new life, but in an astonishing ability to transform, to metamorphosize from one physical identity into another.[16]

In the end, the most salient metamorphosis that Chaplin undertakes is that of the "cinematic body," a body and a performance that is part of the gestalt of the screen, but which also consistently disturbs and disrupts the logic of that screen.

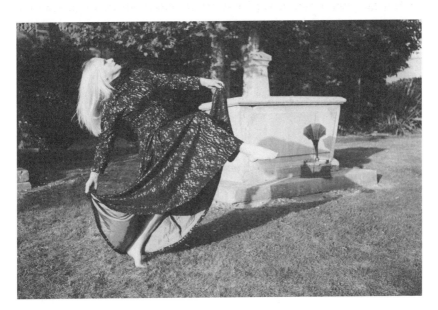

Figure 2.9: *Diva* **(2007) Liz Aggiss**
Liz Aggiss in Diva photo Matthew Andrews

In contemporary screendance, we see this digressive model consistently restated in works such as *Diva*, by Liz Aggiss, a screendance in which we first see her character walking along a red carpet and arriving into the midst of a film shoot. Through the narrative structure and the spoken lines, Aggiss leads us to believe that the film crew is reconstructing a work called "*Largo*," from 1927. We see the method of production and the apparatus of cinema itself in camera, antique gramophone, and so on. There is a close-up of the cameraman's eye seen in reverse through the viewfinder, and then suddenly, the film image shifts to a sepia-toned look in which Aggiss's character embodies a kind of performance quality that suggests we are looking back in time, reflected as well by her costume— a long dress which she manipulates by its hem. The confluence of the surface quality of the media (filmic) and the choreographic language of the performance (historic) results in a scene that is digressive as it veers away from the *present* of the scene that preceded it and seems to move back in time. The scene ends with a close-up of the director's mouth and lips seen through a bullhorn, yelling "cut." We return to the present and a color image as the crew is seen as distracted from the diva's performance, which results in another performance by Aggiss, only this time with a short dress and a more aggressive performance style. This vignette is shot in color and edited with a more contemporary feel. The cuts come more rapidly, and the camera's location changes from shot to shot. Yet, the sound and movement still allude to the silent film ethos of the first sepia-toned section. Aggiss's "balletic-acrobatic-mechanical physical process" is laid bare in *Diva* and further reinforced by the final shot that collapses performer and machine as the Aggiss character leaves the film with the horn of the gramophone slung over her shoulder. *Diva* is thus full of digressive and insurgent moments in the same way that Chaplin's films, punctuated by atemporal swerves, consistently veer away from the master narrative.

Rosalind Krauss further unpacks such narrative disruptions in *The Optical Unconscious* (1993), which offers a history of modernism that defies modernism's "official story," replacing it with one that is full of insurgencies and digressions. She thus encourages a re-reading of official stories, sacred mythologies, and hermetic, self-fulfilling prophesies. It is both interesting and enlightening to apply Krauss's thesis of impurity to the timeline of screendance and, in doing so, resist the modernist tendency toward autonomy and monotheism. By opening up the narrative of screendance to the vast undertaking of modern culture in the first part of the 1900s, we can begin to tell a deeper and more accurate story of the genesis of the form and its subsequent unfolding.

In 1924, for example, René Clair made the film *Entr'acte*, which featured Marcel Duchamp, the enigmatic artist whose larger-than-life presence dominated twentieth-century art history. The film utilizes bodies in motion as well as more recognizable dance vernacular; it is an early example of experimentation with the deconstruction of cinematic space and time via slow-motion movement, superimpositions, and fragmented screen space. Some years later, Maya Deren and Duchamp undertook a project together. In 1943 she began a collaborative film project with Duchamp titled *Witch's Cradle*. Although that film was never completed, it is emblematic of how the diaspora of the visual arts traverses both experimental cinema and dance in the first part of the twentieth century and the modern era, an era marked by a kind of artistic and cultural promiscuity that shows up again in key moments of creativity throughout the century. In this yeasty milieu of collaboration and intermedia experimentation by artists as disparate as Man Ray, René Claire, and Fernand Léger, Marcel Duchamp's gravitational pull intersected with Maya Deren's. The resulting unfinished film offers a glimpse of Deren's early influences as well as some motifs that recur in her more well-known subsequent films, and so serves as further forensic evidence for the link between early screendance and the visual arts. In addition, it begins to flesh out the narrative of the relationship between the visualization of dance on screen and the polyvocal practices of the visual arts since the invention of photography.

The collaboration of Maya Deren and Marcel Duchamp is only one instance of such cross-pollination between modernism and movement.[17] In the first half of the twentieth century both Charlie Chaplin and Buster Keaton were greatly admired by the European Surrealists; the oscillation between the visuality of Surrealism and the vernacular of film is traceable throughout the numerous works of film art that frame dance within the lens—and in particular the works that insert dance into the frame as if it is perfectly natural to do so. The complicating of the performative space with elements of chance encounters becomes evident again in the work of Merce Cunningham many years later; as Roger Copeland pointed out in *What is Dance*, "the goal of dis-unity is to preserve the spectator's perceptual freedom."[18] The dis-unity found in the work of Chaplin and Keaton—the insertion of dance into narrative flow—insists that the viewer not remain passive but aware, sentient, and participatory. This is precisely the kind of phenomena that Krauss pointed to as opposing Greenbergian modernism, along with the kind of agitation from which previous attempts to index the relationship between dance and the camera might benefit.

Modernism and the modern era are rife with contradictions, though. Busby Berkeley, lauded for his deft, highly entertaining combination of dance and film, used dance to enhance the unity of his cinematic spectacles. Like Méliès, Berkeley often used dance as scenic decoration or as a method of enhancing the narrative in his popular films. For example, dancers appear as magical incarnations of shapes and motion, most often shot in deep focus, sometimes from above to amplify movement patterns and spatial designs. The dancers are presented as a part of a highly mechanized, stylized mise-en-scène, typical of the modernist esthetic of the time. The purpose of dance in Berkeley's mechanized spectacles is to draw the viewer's eye to the choreography of large masses of uniform bodies, which are impressive, if only in sheer number. These bodies are ordered by strict spatial configurations that mask individuality and intimacy in favor of reinforcing the power of both cinema and Berkeley himself. Berkeley's dance on film spectacles belong to the general notion of Richard Wagner's *Gesamtkunstwerk*, an integrated space in which all the arts are of equal value. Roger Copeland points out that Bertolt Brecht himself rejected this very sort of practice as one that would "induce sordid intoxication" and one in which "the spectator becomes a passive . . . part of the total work of art."[19] Berkeley's use of dance is a means to an end, the submission of one form to another. But, in the end, Berkeley's dance on screen is a formal exercise that attempts to resist theorizing by sidestepping issues of content in favor of cinematic spectacle.

The films of Maya Deren, in contrast to Berkeley's spectacles and by virtue of their context within the American avant-garde, encourage a more rigorous theoretical inquiry—most notably, her *A Study in Choreography for Camera* (1946), made in collaboration with Talley Beatty. This film has become such a part of the canon of screendance that the actual film itself is often taken for granted and its properties assumed. Where Berkeley's films neutralize the value of the individual, emphasizing instead the importance of the group, Deren's films elevate the individual to a place of power through her use of camera technique and cutting. Where Berkeley's lens dehumanizes, Deren's humanizes and articulates difference in a kind of anti-spectacle. Nevertheless, it is not the formal qualities and concerns of Deren's film ("the leap" so often cited in essays on her work) that are its truly salient aspects; it is rather the insertion of content into form that marks her most important and transgressive contribution to the field. Although the cinematic tricks employed in *A Study* grow out of existing experiments and formal investigations by other filmmakers, and are as such an evolution of form, it is her attention to the dancing body coupled with her surrealist flights of fancy that make this film a pivotal work of screendance.

Most importantly, *A Study* establishes a female-to-male cinematic gaze that is completely at odds with the cinematic practice of the era. In fact, Deren's use of the camera to frame and sexualize the male body precedes by decades discussions about gaze theory and the gendering of cinematic space. In this prescient, political vision, *A Study* stands as a singular work of art. It breaks numerous taboos, transgresses stereotypes, and makes a distinctly political statement by featuring an African American man (Beatty) not as a servant or a butler as Hollywood might have cast him at the time but as a fully formed human being, an elegant and talented dancer, and the sole performer in Deren's four-minute silent film. Beatty's performance is both sensual and sexual, his naked torso suspended in the camera's embrace. Deren's cutting amplifies the intimacy of the viewer's engagement with his image as we track him through both interior and exterior spaces. Deren uses the dancer as the constant in a shifting landscape of place and time, the flow of movement unbroken as location changes from scene to scene, questioning our relationship to the logic of chronology. In addition to the famous unbroken pan, in which we see Beatty in the forest appearing and reappearing as the camera seems to turn 360 degrees on its axis, we also see the dancer begin a gesture in one space and continue it in another seemingly without interruption. In one moment, he moves into a kind of living room where above the mantle we briefly see a framed portrait of Frida Kahlo, a nod to Deren's own proto-feminist identity. In another moment we see Beatty turning on his own axis as the camera frames first torso, then head, then feet, the turning speeding up as the cuts progress. At moments, Beatty seems suspended in midair for an impossible length of time. At other times, an unfolding of the dancer's arm begins in one location and seamlessly ends in another, the choreography literally "moving" the viewer into another place.

In this way, *A Study* is neither abstract nor narrative. Rather, it is "fictive" in the way that Frederick Jameson has used the term to describe the illusion of the passing of already "foreshortened temporalities." Jameson writes that "we all know, but always forget, that the fictive scenes and conversations on the movie screen radically foreshorten reality as the clock ticks and are never . . . coterminous with the putative length of such moments in real life or 'real time.'"[20] Jameson's concept of foreshortened temporalities—cinematic time and space—is at the core of Deren's contribution to screendance. Her film lays the foundation for the deconstruction of the dancing body and its mediatized other as a central principle of screendance. It introduces the viewer to recorporealization, the complete construction of an impossible cinematic body, in which the real and the fictive are hybridized. Simultaneously, she creates a work of art in which dance, removed from narrative responsibility, is contingent on neither what precedes it nor what follows it in the frame. In thinking about film anagrammatically, Deren explains:

> In an anagram all the elements exist in a simultaneous relationship. . . . Each element of an anagram is so related to the whole that no one of them may be changed without affecting its series and so affecting the whole. And conversely the whole is so related to every part that whether one reads horizontally, vertically, diagonally or even in reverse, the logic of the whole is not disrupted, but remains intact.[21]

A Study in Choreography for Camera illustrates Deren's ideas about the anagrammatic possibilities of screendance, while the dancer, screenically inscribed, is both the subject and the object of the camera's gaze, estheticized and recorporealized.

Deren's work at the intersection of theory and practice preceded and catalyzed countless mediated representations of dance. An inheritor of Deren's proto-feminist legacy, Yvonne Rainer is claimed equally by the dance and experimental film communities, and as such, the transition of Rainer from dance maker to filmmaker in 1972 (and back to dance maker in 2000) embodies the porous membranes of both dance and media practices. Although Rainer worked in film, the theoretical groundwork for a relationship between dance and its mediated other was laid in the liminal state between the heady days of experimental film in the 1960s and the coming of age of video technology later in that decade. This relationship was inexorably tied to the advent of postmodernism and, by extension, *video* culture.

In 1972 Rainer made the film *Lives of Performers*, bringing her choreographic sensibility with her and creating a hybrid style that made her a force in avant-garde film circles. Erin Brannigan notes:

> What links Rainer's dance and film work is an intense critique of disciplinary conventions and a profound interrogation of the role of performance. Performance is central to all aspects of Rainer's work; she herself refers to performance as the subject matter in her films.[22]

Rainer is a pivotal figure in the landscape of screendance for a number of reasons, and she physically embodied the shift in dance from modern to postmodern. As Sally Banes points out, "in early postmodern dance, the performers . . . did not 'perform' or even represent emotion in terms of character, narrative or even abstraction." The dancers "reveled in the matter-of-factness of ordinary movement found in the performance of tasks and other everyday activities." In doing so, "postmodern dance shifted the long-standing debate in dance theory about whether dance should be an art of expression or of technical virtuosity to a new key, because it valued neither." Instead, Banes observes that "it opted for the dance as a frame to scrutinize movement-action-as material." The idea of dance as a "frame" has obvious connotations for Rainer's migration from the movement of dance to the moving image of film. Banes's description of "dance as a frame to scrutinize movement-action-as material" might be reworked to read "the *frame as a site* to scrutinize movement-action-as material."[23] By slightly reordering Banes's notion of dance as the frame, we can shift the site of the "scrutinizing" to camera space, marking it as a site to scrutinize, excavate, and illuminate movement ideas in the space of video, the digital, or electronic landscape that Rainer makes possible in such films as *Lives of Performers* and *Film About a Woman Who*.

While Rainer's work has been situated in the context of new scholarship on performance by scholars like Peggy Phelan and Erin Brannigan, it is important to note that Rainer's work is also *visual*. It is inscribed as film within a visual culture. Although working in film at the time, her trajectory away from liveness and toward the mediation of dance is a blueprint for screendance in general. Brannigan writes:

> In *Lives of Performers* there is no higher order or purpose structuring the action on screen and the elements and sections of the film are strung together like her uninflected dance phrases; no single part is given more value, the score is not subservient to the visuals, there is no central character with whom we identify.[24]

What Brannigan describes is a liminal state in which Rainer's work is perched on the threshold of a new model as she leaves behind the form of dance and adopts the form of cinema. This blurring of boundaries creates a genre that most represents the nascent (in 1972) forms of *performance art* and *video art*. There is certainly ample evidence to speak of her work solely in terms of avant-garde film. The references to Futurist, Dadaist, and Surrealist movements seem clear as well, references also shared by the first wave of video artists such as Nam June Paik, whose work similarly blurs the boundaries of media, performance, and the visual arts. While materially Rainer made work in 1972 in the medium of film, her methodology coincides with, and in some cases precedes, artists' use of video as a site for arranging numerous ideas and actions that do not rely on traditional rules of engagement. The work functions in much the same way that other artists at the time—Martha Rosler and Vito Acconci for example—used *video* to dislocate narrative and to insert first-person identity into the frame. As Rainer's work is most often situated in film, its unnamable genre (dance, film, cine-dance?) represents the uncertainty and polyvocality that marks postmodern art practices, or more specifically marks the liminal stage between modernism and postmodernism, the very space from which screendance emerges in the coming era of video.

CHAPTER 3

Recorporealization and the Mediated Body

Contemporary life is a mix of simulated, mediatized, analog and digital, flesh and machine, and often the delineations between these states are unrecognizable. That we live in a collaged culture is a given. The deconstruction, reconstruction, and hybridization of the detritus of culture, and the ephemeral and immaterial traces of experience, is a methodology that traverses the entire twentieth century and continues to the present. From the cinematic montages of Eisenstein and Vertov to the collages of Max Ernst, Kurt Schwitters, and the Surrealists, through Duchamp and Warhol, modernism's path toward ascetic reductivism is littered with photographic images. Such images undermine modernism's trajectory toward minimalism or at least keep it "real" in the way that the art critic Hal Foster refers to a grounding in actual bodies and social sites.[1] Subsequently, as postmodernism has moved inexorably toward digital culture and as mediated images of bodies in motion become more and more ubiquitous, from YouTube to digital billboards, screendance as a site of practice aligns itself with the histories and theories of mediation in a number of ways.

Dancing bodies perform a particular kind of logic, choreographic, kinesthetic, or otherwise. Even considering the possibilities of virtuosic performance made possible by contemporary training methodologies, human bodies performing in real time and space are constrained by both somatic and temporal absolutes ➒. When bodies move in ways that are beyond such absolutes, bones break, muscles tear, and, in general, the body is subject to corporeal havoc or a kind of annihilation. Mediated images of bodies in motion are subject to a different sort of logic, one that is without the corporeal terror that is wrought by tearing, effacing, reordering, and stitching

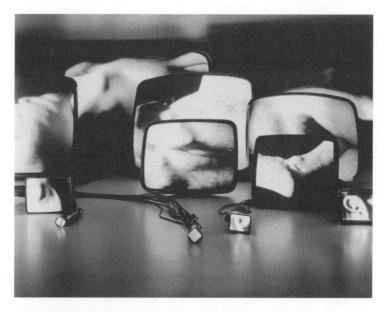

Figure 3.2: Inasmuch as It Is Already Taking Place (1990), Gary Hill
GARY HILL Inasmuch As It Is Always Already Taking Place, 1990 – Detail Sixteen-channel video/sound installation
Sixteen modified 1/2-inch to 23-inch black-and-white video monitors (cathode ray tubes removed from chassis), two speakers, sixteen DVD players and sixteen DVDs (black-and-white; one with stereo sound)
Dimensions of horizontal niche: 16 h. x 54 x 66 in. (41 x 137 x 167 cm.)
Edition of two and one artist's proof
PHOTO CREDIT: Mark B. McLoughlin, Courtesy of the artist and Donald Young Gallery, Chicago

together fragments of movement or body parts that do not logically flow in such an arrangement. The author and critic Rebecca Solnit refers to the "instruments for 'annihilating time and space'"—including the telephone, photography, and the railroad—as the beginning of the "modern world," and she notes that cinema offers a "breach in the wall between the past and the present."[2] While speeding trains certainly put our relationship to time and space in a new perspective, in the post-cinema, digital era, such annihilation can be accomplished by simply transposing the order of simultaneous frames of digital media. The ease by which a violent unhinging of linear time can be accomplished in digital media is a continuation of modern cinema's predilection for compressing time and space into its own system of narrative logic, one that limits the marks of inscription *to* the body while migrating further inscription to the material of recording and mediation.

While nonlinearity and fragmentation are recognizable traits of post-modernism in general, art created in the postmodern era is not monolithic, and the tension between the desire for a certain kind of time-space logic, often found in choreographic practice, can collide with a desire for a reorganization of time and space in mediated representations of choreographic ideas. Screendance questions the way in which choreographic ideas *in practice* are historically and typically corporealized. Re-siting the choreographic impulse within the material space of media offers a considerable spectrum of possibilities, each more or less representational and/or contingent on the qualities of dance in real time and space.

At one end of this spectrum is documentation: the recording of a live dance performance. At the opposite end of the spectrum is screendance: the articulation of choreographic ideas completely contingent on the specificities of media space. It is at this end of the spectrum where ideas about the body can be unmoored from somatic and corporeal absolutes, where bodies can be re-imagined and, yes, *re*corporealized. Recorporealization refers to the literal reconstruction of the dancing body via screen techniques; at times a construction of an impossible body, one not encumbered by gravity, temporal restraints, or death.

In order to recorporealize the body, however, it must first be *de*-corporealized, and ideas about corporeality must also be interrogated. Corporeality implies physicality, materiality, and a contingency on the nature of the body. Conceptually, it conjures images of the body in the flesh, adhering to somatic boundaries and a kind of natural order.

Eadweard Muybridge's motion studies provide a template for a mediated representation of the performing body, which is illustrative of how media may be used to preserve corporeality and, at the same time, prove its limits in time and space. Muybridge's image sets consistently flow from past to present, illustrating (and preceding) the linearity of cinematic logic. The bodies in his studies generally perform an action from start to finish—for example, a man walks up a set of stairs, a woman walks across the floor and bends to pick up an object, or the arc of the task performed is framed as beginning and ending by the camera's recording. There are no disturbances or disruptions to corporeality in his image sets; rather, they function as proofs of a tendency toward order in human movement and its subsequent mediation.

Akira Mizuta Lippit notes in his essay "Digesture," that "Movement is measured in time and captured in cinema, a feature unavailable in still photography. Unlike photography, which preserves only the body as such, cinema preserves an image of the body in motion."[3] However, the act of preservation that Lippit describes only forestalls the possibility of

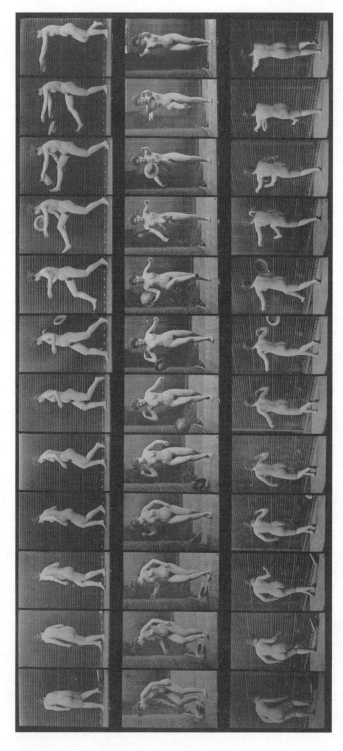

Figure 3.3: Eadweard Muybridge *Woman. Kicking*. Plate 367 from Animal Locomotion. 1887. Collotype, 7 1/2x20 ¼". Gift of the Philadelphia Commercial Museum. The Museum of Modern Art/Licensed by SCALA/Art Resource, NY

remediating such images. In other words, the *moment* of a body in motion that might be preserved is only preserved *for* the moment. The very gesture of its preservation creates the possibility that such moments may be recorporealized into a kind of screenic body in motion, not of the cinema and its histories but rather of the screen and its specificities. Such preserved moments of screenic movement are the material by which one may undo the photographic, linear representation of bodies in motion and recalculate on screen the potentials both virtual and metaphoric of such bodies. Screendance thus, as it *undoes* the temporal nature of "choreography," recorporealizes the bodies it represents and also rematerializes those bodies as a hybrid that is both corporeal and mediated. Thus, the decorporealization (the undoing) of screenic bodies necessarily precedes their recorporealization.

While optical technologies present the possibility of a faithful or realistic representation of the body, screendance pivots on images of bodies that are *re*-presented and recorporealized in order to create a new lexicon of movement-based images. Situating movement within the architecture of the camera—camera space—and its relative technological possibilities allows for an exploration of and a re-imagining of the metaphoric and poetic possibilities of the body. However, the relationship of bodies to the technologies of representation, of recording and of re-ordering, is complicated and diverse. Lippit suggests that such representations within camera space are a kind of "erasure of bodies in the world," and that the "movements that are produced as an effect of the apparatus . . . are defined prosthetically." Their inscription is thus made possible and further, made *by* the apparatus of filmmaking.[4]

Since the emergence of the optical mediums as a means of representation, the body has played a significant role in the development of such technologies and their subsequent uses. While painters had long focused their gaze on the body, a significant turning point in the relationship between representation, artistic practice, and perception arrived with the advent of photography in the mid-nineteenth century. Michael Rush reminds us, in *New Media in Late Twentieth-Century Art*, that "from the beginnings of photography . . . art and technology co-existed in an essential bond that has benefited both for more than one hundred years."[5] In the same way that the *camera obscura* influenced Italian and Dutch Renaissance painters and the lithograph affected the reproduction and distribution of art images, the invention of photography caused art and technology to engage in a vigorous interaction. Photography freed artists from the obligation of documenting life via painting, opening up a wide expanse of possibilities in art making. Photography, as it was embraced by the

Futurists, the Dada movement, and others, influenced how new paintings were created: rather than attempting to accurately reflect the objective world, artists began to create images that embodied somatic experience and spatial relationships.

Works such as Marcel Duchamp's *Nude Descending a Staircase, No. 2* (1912) strongly reflected the influence of the photograph; more specifically they referenced the "chronophotography" of Etienne-Jules Marey and motion studies of Eadweard Muybridge. According to Margot Lovejoy, the experiments of Marey and others, "served as inspiration for the Cubists and Futurists, who were directly influenced by the broken, serialized abstract linear patterns of movement."[6] Technologies of the moving image as developed in the early 1900s enabled artists to explore multiple frames of reference and take advantage of the fluidity of cinematic time. While the

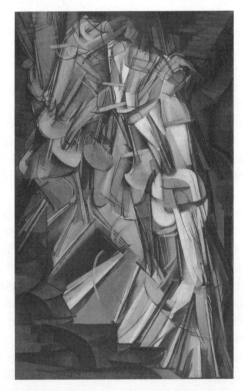

Figure 3.4: *Nude Descending a Staircase, No. 2* **(1912), Marcel Duchamp**
Accession #1950-134-59 Nude Descending a Staircase (No. 2) Marcel Duchamp Oil on canvas, 1912
57 7/8 x 35 1/8 inches (147 x 89.2 cm)
Philadelphia Museum of Art: The Louise and Walter Arensberg Collection, 1950
© 2010 Artists Rights Society (ARS), New York/ADAGP, Paris/Succession Marcel Duchamp

Russian filmmaker Sergei Eisenstein, an artist with training in engineering, mathematics, and art, perfected the techniques of film editing and cinematic montage, he owed much of his varied camera angle work and sophisticated editing to "the fragmented shapes of Cubism, in which multiple views of reality . . . allowed for multiple understandings of reality."[7]

The specificity of camera space offers a range of possibilities in which boundaries begin to dissolve, overlaps occur, and lateral shifts in understanding and in the representations of bodies take may hold. It is in this liminal space, the space between the architecture of the theater and the "real" landscape, that the fragmentary possibilities of photographic representation make it possible to see movement atemporally, its minutiae made visible. And as culture becomes more and more mediatized, our eyes begin to see differently and perception shifts accordingly. Here is a point of tangency between photographic representation and screendance, where the spheres of contemporary dance and contemporary art overlap, and hybrid forms emerge. Photographic image-moments often function most effectively in groups. A single photograph, while potentially powerful in and of itself, offers us no past and no future. It is "out of time," so to speak. An accretion of photographic evidence via multiple images creates a situation in which one image contextualizes another, and so on, until a particular logic or at least a trajectory of some sort becomes apparent. Eadweard Muybridge's motion studies hinged upon such a logic: past, present, and future within a single frame. And this logic is the phenomenon that screendance is predicated on as well. The accretion of isolated moments of bodies in motion, suspended on film or as digital information, is often without context (when each frame is considered on its own), and so content or meaning is obscured. But when these isolated image-moments are brought together into a montage, collisions occur, as do juxtapositions that directly affect the perception of somatic and kinesthetic qualities as well as the ultimate meaning of such work.

While meaning in photography generally emerges from discrete images, screendance relies on a sequential accretion of similar images. The leap from photography to screendance, then, is not as great as it might seem: both share a number of historical and theoretical narratives. Particular modes of postmodern representation overlap both photography and screendance, and also illuminate and further contextualize screendance itself. Specifically, the screendance that is recognizable for its deconstructivist, fragmentary representation of the body, its reliance on altered temporality, and its contingent screenic sensibility is a product of the evolution of a technological/theoretical dialectic that reached its apex the end of the twentieth century.

Between the end of abstract expressionism's heyday and the resurgence of painting in the 1980s, the landscape of contemporary art (including dance) underwent considerable upheaval. Subsequent to the 1958 death of abstract expressionism's most prominent practitioner, Jackson Pollock, the artist Allen Kaprow published his prophetic essay, *The Legacy of Jackson Pollock*. Kaprow sensed that Pollock's death opened a door to a new way of experiencing the world and put forth his thoughts as a kind of prognostication.

> Pollock, as I see him, left us at the point where we must become preoccupied with, and even dazzled by the space and objects of our everyday life, either our bodies, clothes, rooms, or, if need be, the vastness of Forty-Second Street. Not satisfied with the suggestion through paint of our other senses, we shall utilize the specific substances of sight, sound, movements, people, odors, touch. Objects of every sort are materials for this new art: paint, chairs, food, electric and neon lights, smoke, water, old socks, a dog, movies, a thousand other things that will be discovered by the present generation of artists. . . . An odor of crushed strawberries, a letter from a friend, or a billboard selling Drano; three taps on the front door, a scratch, a sigh, or a voice lecturing endlessly . . . all will become materials for this new concrete art. . . . Young artists of today need no longer say, "I am a painter" or "a poet" or "a dancer". They are simply "artists."[8]

Kaprow's essay was a virtual mantra for all areas of art practice, and it seeped into dance through practitioners such as Simone Forti, Anna Halprin, and Yvonne Rainer. At that time, according to Sally Banes in *Terpsichore in Sneakers*, "The new theater, like the new visual art, was in a process of dematerialization. . . . Allan Kaprow's Happenings set precedents for breakdowns between art and life experiences."[9] The dematerialization of disciplinary boundaries and the politics of postmodernism were undertaken by the dance world—notably by the Judson Church Dance Theater choreographers in New York—forever altering and rupturing the forward motion of modern dance by opening the practice outward to embrace film and ideas about materiality and temporality more often associated with the visual arts.

Banes's allusion to the writer Lucy Lippard's ideas about "dematerialization" in the frame of postmodern dance is not inconsequential. As Lippard notes, speaking about conceptual art of the late 1960s:

> [A] number of new subjects and approaches appeared: narrative, role-playing, guise and disguise, body and beauty issues; a focus on fragmentation,

interrelationships, autobiography, performance, daily life, and of course on feminist politics.[10]

In the moment of cultural upheaval that straddled the decade of 1960s and 1970s, various factions of the art world cross-pollinated to such an extent that at times, one previously recognizable discipline simply morphed into another.[11] The idea of media, performance, theater, and even objects became fluid, the various viscosities of each discipline allowing for a kind of mixing-bowl effect that still resonates in the contemporary practice of screendance. Perhaps more than anything, though, it was performance and its offspring that most dramatically altered the landscape.

The term "performance art" came into being in the 1970s as a way of contextualizing and separating an artist's performance from experimental theater and the Happenings of the 1950s and 1960s. The rise of performance as an art-making practice parallels the unfolding of feminism in the United States and owes much of its ideology to feminist practice and discourse. Making the personal political, an idea born out of feminism, offered a way for performance artists to speak about deeply personal issues and, at the same time, connect those issues with larger social ones. The performance art of the 1970s, coming on the heels of conceptualism and minimalism, was very much about process, about setting a task and engaging in the ritual of accomplishing it. Much of the work was done in complete privacy and known later only through its documentation. For example, in Eleanor Antin's *Carving, (8 days) A Traditional Sculpture*, 1972, made from July 15, 1972, to August 21, 1972, the artist was photographed every morning over the course of forty-five days as she followed a strict weight-loss diet. This performance and its mediation questions both the traditional notion of sculpture as well as the production of an ideal body as prescribed by the culture. Note the fragmented, durational, and almost cinematic representation of Antin's changing body and the unmistakable echoes of Eadweard Muybridge's motion studies in the documentation.

Many of performance artist Chris Burden's pieces, including *Shoot* and *Five Day Locker Piece*, both from 1971, and *Trans-fixed* (1974) were also known primarily through their photographic documentation. Artists such as Adrian Piper and Vito Acconci made work in public spaces that was often unannounced until after the work was realized. At times, no one but the artists knew a performance was taking place, and in fact much early performance work eschewed audiences, instead relying on mediated images of the event in the form of video, film, or photographs that served as a kind of proof of their existence.

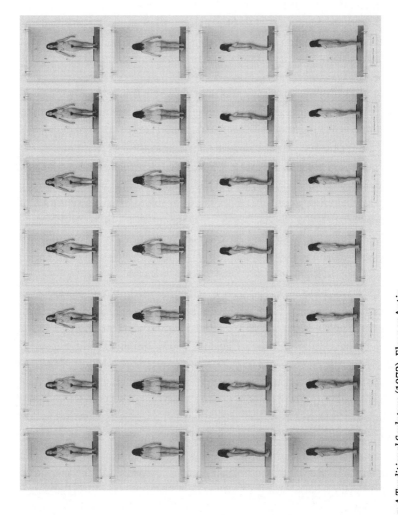

Figure 3.5: *Carving: A Traditional Sculpture* (1972), Eleanor Antin
"The Last Seven Days" from *Carving: A Traditional Sculpture*, 1972/99 28 gelatin silver prints with labels and wall texteach: 7 x 5 inches
Courtesy Ronald Feldman Fine Arts, New York"

Photographs (as well as videotape of the same era), especially film-based, black and white prints or reprints, had the aura of authenticity about them.[12] They situated the work of early performance art in a particular time frame, contingent on a particular technology as their means of currency. The grainy, degraded look of photography and video of the era ironically became, then, one of its most recognizable traits, a visual cue that suggested that what had occurred was, in fact, real. Such documentation created a palpable sense of the moment, unadorned and decidedly nontheatrical. The tools of documentation used to mark the existence of ephemeral performance work of the era were the same tools that were increasingly found in the homes and hands of non-artists as well. As technology began to democratize access to such image-making tools by making them simpler, cheaper, and more accessible, the space between "artist" and "non-artist" collapsed. And the space in which mediated images were produced and distributed began to considerably diminish. This diminishment further manifested itself as a collapsing of the space between art and life, setting the stage for a particular kind of evolutionary thinking about art in general, including Allan Kaprow's ideas about "life-like art" and "art-like art."[13]

"Art-like art," Kaprow said, could be easily recognized in relation to all that preceded it. In other words, we can recognize a sculpture or a painting specifically because it looks like other sculpture and painting. Art-like art is further contextualized by its location, generally in a museum or gallery. What Kaprow proposed was a radical rethinking of the nature of art and art practices, or "life-like art." Kaprow suggested eliminating all theatrical convention as well as art contexts, including audiences, "single time/place envelopes," narrative, acting skills, rehearsals, and repeated performances.[14] After arriving at that conclusion, the next leap was to recognize alternative actions that might be considered as performance, such as brushing your teeth, washing dishes, talking to a friend, and so on. The Happenings of the 1950s, which Kaprow initiated and named, were grounded in events occurring in real time. Kaprow writes, "Doing life, consciously, was a compelling notion to me."[15] Kaprow referred to this new genre as art/life, his attempt to meld life with art. The notion that art could come directly out of one's life experience held numerous possibilities for artists intent on creating performative work and using increasingly more accessible, everyday tools of representation as a means of circulating the traces of such work. By extension, screendance offered the possibility of fusing moving image technologies with the technologies and techniques of dance or movement. Such mediation of real bodies in motion, was placed within the technologies of the era and resulted in an art form that echoed

Kaprow's call for a recognition of the real. While it could be argued that representations of dance on film or video are not "real" in any number of definitions, the process by which actual bodies in motion are inscribed on film, video, or contemporary digital technologies is in itself the actual recording of a performed moment or gesture.

As photography and film technologies became an inextricable part of twentieth-century culture, it enabled a greater reliance on image as a mnemonic device for memory.[16] And in this shift, memory underwent a transition not only in form but in function as well. The well-known art critic John Berger asks:

> What served in place of the photograph before the camera's invention? The expected answer is the engraving, the drawing, the painting. The more revealing answer might be: memory. What photographs do out there in space was previously done within reflection. . . . Yet, unlike memory, photographs do not in themselves preserve meaning. They offer appearances—with all the credibility and gravity we normally lend to appearances prised away from their meanings.[17]

Extending Berger's comments, we might say that as the optical and reproductive technologies that make photography possible become more transparent, memory is liberated. Given a photograph, for example, our need to remember is diminished. However, the need to *contextualize* the traces that a photograph preserves becomes greater. Photographs and their afterimages, the ephemera and shards offering clues of an event or action that has occurred, have played an integral part in the construction of a modern culture, which has come to value photographic evidence as a marker for human experience. A photograph implies that something has happened. The photographic process has long been relied upon to document and comment on both quotidian and more spectacular cultural phenomena. From the earliest days of photography and its ghostly traces of people and places, through the socially conscious work of activists such as Jacob Riis to the Hollywood-inspired pictures of Cindy Sherman, photographed images have actively shaped culture.

As performative work increased in cultural value in the 1970s and '80s, dance began to focus on the possibilities for archiving its histories, enabled by new, high-quality, consumer-grade video equipment. Such video recording equipment, of lower cost and higher quality, made it possible for choreographers in the 1980s to attain reasonably accurate recordings of their performances. Prior to this, much of the earliest modern dance was recorded only in hard-to-access films or in notation form. Given the scarcity and limitations of retrievable or re-viewable mediated representations of early modern dance, the mythologies surrounding such work have increased. In the age of video reproduction, however, dance began to document itself incessantly; the resulting documentation serves both as a reminder to the choreographer, a way to recuperate the work and also as currency in the more pragmatic aspects of the business of dance, such as funding applications and performance opportunities. Thus, documentation has sought to preserve the choreographer's work in total: as a hedge against cultural erasure and the vagaries of memory. Screendance applies the technologies of representation to a different set of desires, with different outcomes and expectations.

Dancing bodies perform a kind of automatic writing: in space it is ephemeral, but on film and video the "text" is reified and actualized. Maya Deren's *A Study in Choreography for Camera* (chap. 2) is an apt example of a filmmaker "writing" with film in a way that enables both *recuperation* and *recorporealization*. Deren's use of the camera and subsequent editing of the filmed moments are performative in the most literal sense of the word: they are virtual utterances that negate the received cultural meaning of the black male body, rewriting it in screenic space. Through the film's montage of landscape and the juxtaposition of meaningful symbols, Deren crafts a nonlinear, abstract narrative that recuperates the dignity and sexuality of the dancer Talley Beatty which had been previously eviscerated by racist culture (Beatty is a stand-in for all people of color in the pre-civil rights era). Art, culture, and beauty conspire with the stunning presence of Beatty's dancing and Deren's camerawork to enable a radical cinematic transformation. Deren rewrites and simultaneously "rights" the prevailing culture as she recorporealizes Beatty's dancing body into one capable of expanded physicality. It is simultaneously a fiction and a promise of the possibility of film to articulate the metaphors of bodies in motion.

In *Nine Variations on a Dance Theme* (1967), the director Hilary Harris extends Deren's vision by achieving a composition in which the dance and the film are inextricable: both are part of a gestalt in which neither can be seen if not through the lens of the other. Harris identified the potential in the overlap of dance and film, for an unexplored area in which one could create kinesthetic and cinematic poetry. This poetry relied on a densely conceptual, structural approach to composition. What is particularly interesting about *Nine Variations*, however, is that whether intentionally or inadvertently, Harris interrogates the illusionary power of film to recorporealize a dancing body from its cinematic corpus. *Nine Variations on a Dance Theme* (shot and edited by Harris) with the dancer Bettie de Jong

performing, is at first glance conceptually straightforward: a short movement phrase (fifty seconds) by De Jong is performed in the same way nine
different times. It then is interpreted through shot composition and editing, in nine different ways, by Harris. The film is shot in a loft-like space
with a window on one wall and no decoration or props in the camera's view.
Throughout the film it is evident that individual shots are made at different
times of the day and in different seasons by the changing quality of the
natural luminosity that lights the space. As Harris's film begins, we see
De Jong dancing a lyrical phrase from an objective distance—that is to say
we see her framed in a wide shot, the camera locked down, unmoving,
her arms carving space and finally spiraling to the floor. At the beginning of
the film, the dancer articulates movement across the plane of the camera's
lens. As the film progresses, a subtle shift occurs where the camera begins
to move in opposition or counterpoint to the dancer. The result is an accu-
mulation of compound angles, serendipitous encounters in which a hand
crosses the screen, a foot comes to rest, the curve of the body moves
away from the arc of the moving camera. Another complication is added
when Harris's editing increases in rapidity: the cuts come faster, and the
material is deconstructed and reconstructed before the viewer's eye until
the movement phrase and De Jong's dancing body have been completely
recorporealized into a fragmented, sutured version of the original opening
shot.[18]

Roland Barthes writes:

> Where is your authentic body? You are the only one who can never see yourself
> except as an image; you never see your eyes unless they are dulled by the gaze
> they rest upon the mirror or the lens . . . even and especially for your own body,
> you are condemned to the repertoire of its images.[19]

Barthes pondered his own authenticity while gazing at images of himself.
Such a gesture is often repeated in the creation of screendance as
movement is performed, recorded and replayed. If authenticity is to be
considered as one desired outcome or end point for a work of art, including
screendance, then what is authentic about *Nine Variations* and, further,
what is authentic about the body at the center of the film?

Hilary Harris, in his function as photographer and editor of De Jong's
dancing body, exercises considerable auteurship in regard to the "repertoire
of . . . images" to which Barthes refers. Literally inscribing the trace of
De Jong's physicality and corporeality onto the surface of film, Harris
shot the footage for *Nine Variations* in some twenty-five sessions, averag-
ing two or three hours each over a period of one year. The body we see on

film is a different body than the one that De Jong stretched and moved in real time and space; that is, it is not the body of De Jong on a particular day in 1967 but a body constructed over the course of a year, and a body that was in the process of becoming itself as it was being rendered on film. Sally Ann Ness observes:

> The dancer's body can be seen to form the "host material," a living tissue for dance's gestural inscriptions. Its anatomy provides the "sites" or "places" where gesture can leave its mark in the rendering of a "final form"—that is in a structure that bears an enduring and permanent signifying character ⬤.[20]

If, as Ness proposes, the body itself is a site of inscription, "the host material," then there is a doubling of such as the film also inscribes and reinscribes the body's gestural presence. The process of becoming, of aging, of maturing, is all fixed within *Nine Variations*, though what we ultimately see is a lyrical, kinetic, and highly edited version of a dancing body—an impossible body, a recorporealized body in the "final form" of the film.

All the while, the filmed version augurs for its own authenticity. Harris intentionally decorporealizes her performance and recorporealizes it into a new construction; out of the conspiracy of cinematic technique and De Jong's performance, Harris creates a new kind of authenticity, one that is a hybrid of performance and technological intervention. According to Walter Benjamin, in photography, even "the tiniest authentic fragment of daily life" has the potential to convey volumes. In pondering the place of authenticity in art generally, he notes for instance, that "the revolutionary strength of Dadaism consisted in testing art for its authenticity."[21] For Benjamin, authentic things were real things, the detritus of culture, a cigarette butt, a spool of cotton. Put in a frame, these things "rupture time" and move toward photomontage, which, for Benjamin, was a revolutionary form. But what is authentic about *Nine Variations*? It is clearly a construction of disparate parts, sleight of hand, and impossible phenomena. At the same time, though, it is an accretion of images that are clearly "real," almost journalistic. While the provenance of the choreography may be of a particular modern dance lineage, the movement is embodied, the effort clear, and the performance undeniable. In the process of articulating a screendance, authenticity migrates from the "live" performative body to the archive of film or video. In this migration, the corporeal body is shed like snakeskin, its usefulness finished, its image inscribed, its absence leaving a permanent yet ephemeral inscription of its performance. The result is a recollection, a screen memory that is now both the mnemonic for those days in 1967 when De Jong performed for Harris's camera and the referent of her corporeality.

Maya Deren's and Hilary Harris's films may indeed serve as models that represent the maturation of a unique engagement with the body through screendance, in which the body is raw material for a reconceptualization of corporeality; in which mechanical reproduction recorporealizes the body; and in which the filmed, edited body becomes the authentic body as it outlives its subject. This methodology arguably privileges the director, and yet it can also provide an opportunity for the dancer to author her own autobiography and self-representation. In the case of Bettie de Jong, in Harris's *Nine Variations*, by subjecting herself to a year of shooting and repeatedly dancing the same phrase over and over, she insures through mechanical reproduction that she is immune from the effacement or absence that comes with the end of a dancer's *dancing* life. And in the case of Talley Beatty, his image on film, even subsequent to Deren's manipulation, or perhaps because of it, maintains its desire and inscribes a particular and specific performance of self-representation.

Screendance is thus a process of both inscription and effacement. As the work of screendance comes into being, from shooting through editing, its *original* is gradually effaced. The effacement is largely realized in the editing process when individual shots, the "text" of the dance, are hacked off the body of material inscribed in film or as digital data and jettisoned as the editor creates a new logic and recorporealizes the dancing bodies. In digital editing, this process is made even more metaphorically real, as chunks of material (the corpus) are dragged to the "trash" and leave behind no trace of their existence.[22]

The dance critic John Martin theorized that dance (especially modern dance) was an art of expression; he uses the term "metakinesis" to describe the situation in which the viewer is drawn into the dance. Martin states, "Because of the inherent contagion of bodily movement, which makes the onlooker feel sympathetically in his own musculature, the dancer is able to convey through movement the most intangible emotional experience."[23] The parallel in screendance to the "inherent contagion" that Martin describes as metakinesis may be thought of as a *kinestronic* response—the combination or merging of the kinesthetic and electronic. In the screen version of a dance, a trace of Martin's inherent contagion remains. However, the sympathetic emotional experience he describes is, in the mediated dance, exacerbated and further articulated by camera techniques, and also by the maker's ability to frame issues of loss, pain, identity, and so forth within a recognizable form.

The "most intangible emotional experience" the dancer is able to convey through metakinesis is made all the more potent in the screendance with the addition of first-person narrative, the use of the close-up to add intimacy, the sound of the dancers' breaths, and editing techniques, all of which allow the makers to cite or acknowledge what is particular to the possibilities of the moving image, adding depth to the narrative or text of the work, metaphors of place, memory, and site, encouraging the viewer to feel a kinestronic response. In a screendance, Martin's "most intangible emotional experience" may be inscribed in film or video and is recoverable through viewing at any given time, thus recuperating the ephemeral image and experience.[24]

The camera catalyzes a reverence for the dance and focuses the act of seeing in a way that is quite different than the perceptual act that one might practice as a matter of habit. *Camera-looking* is an active performance that frames an event and elevates it while "screening out" all other information.[25] It is an act that implies a reverence for that which is framed and eschews all that is outside the frame. In doing so it parses activity into essential and nonessential, absent and present, and presupposes the editing process—which further parses individual moments of mediated performance into even smaller partitions. One would suppose that the mediation of live dance by a recording device would distance the viewer from the activity framed. The opposite occurs, however, for the cameraperson as she engages the dancer within the frame. The phenomenon is one in which the camera becomes a prosthetic for seeing and often, in the experience of the cameraperson, transforms the ordinary into the extraordinary.

Through this vision-prosthetic, a very particular kind of intimacy is created between the camera operator and the performer, something sensual and of the flesh. It is a metaphor that has been noted by numerous theorists, including Roland Barthes, who states, "A sort of umbilical cord links the body of the photographed thing to my gaze: light, though impalpable, is here a carnal medium, a skin I share with anyone who has been photographed."[26] The act of recorporealization implies a kind of flesh and blood reanimation. It calls to mind Frankensteinian narratives in which flesh is flayed open, repaired and re-authored: embodied in the intimate relationship between the surgeon and patient, and the subsequent corporeal alchemy. Again, to return to Benjamin:

> The magician heals a sick person by the laying on of hands; the surgeon cuts into the patient's body. The magician maintains the natural distance between the patient and himself; though he reduces it very slightly by the laying on of hands,

he greatly increases it by virtue of his authority. The surgeon does exactly the reverse; he greatly diminishes the distance between himself and the patient by penetrating into the patient's body, and increases it but little by the caution with which his hand moves among the organs. In short, in contrast to the magician—who is still hidden in the medical practitioner—the surgeon at the decisive moment abstains from facing the patient man to man; rather, it is through the operation that he penetrates into him.[27]

As Benjamin notes, eschewing face-to-face contact, it is through "the operation" that the surgeon penetrates his subject. In the creation of a screendance, the theater of operations is not unlike the operating room: the surgeon cuts into the patient's body, the camera operator cuts the patient/dancer's body, both metaphorically and literally, by cropping the frame to dissect limbs and motion, virtually fragmenting and deconstructing the body. It is a bloodless amputation but an amputation nonetheless, a prelude to the further cutting that will occur in the postproduction process as the body is recorporealized. Face-to-face contact is impaired in the recording of movement, made impossible by the mediation that occurs as the camera operator gazes at the dancer through the lens, a separation that is made even more evident when viewing the process on a discrete screen or monitor. The parallels between medical intervention and the production of a screendance go even deeper if one considers that many medical procedures are viewed by the surgeon and her assistants on screens placed around the operating theater. The body in surgery is mediated by live video feeds from cameras both outside and inside the body, and recorporealization of the body is accomplished via video simulation or representation.

The spectacle that one encounters in Benjamin's surgical theater is not unlike the spectacle of a film or video shoot. In the case of the surgeon and that of the camera operator, the method of production is necessarily absent in the final product, though its inscription remains as a trace. The body is stitched up, wheeled out of the operating theater, and sent on its way. The mediatized body of the dancer is recorporealized, rendered whole again, though not without a kind of permanent, metaphoric wound, and inscribed in the embrace of film or the digital environment. The wound left on the recorporealized body is the phantom pain of that which is amputated by the frame of the camera and the editing process: bits of movement, an arm, a leg, the connective tissue that previously bound together the logic of choreography made in real time.

Benjamin's "magic," or more particularly a sort of ritual that ends in magical transformation, is present both in the case of the surgeon and in the production of the screendance. Each requires a deliberate, focused, and methodical set of procedures. And each requires a deep faith in the outcome of those procedures that resembles, at least formally, a belief in magic and the kind of corporeal transformation that mechanical reproduction has enabled. The magic alluded to by Benjamin can be seen in another light as well. The migration of dance from its live, corporeal performance to a simulation of itself in film or digital technologies is contingent *on* alchemy. The notion of turning one thing into another is a staple of alchemical fantasy, but in the creation of a screendance it is more than simple fantasy. The "magic of cinema" notwithstanding, the ability to recorporealize dancing bodies into digital data, while not technically magic, certainly flows from a similar metaphor.

In John Sanborn and Mary Perillo's video piece *Untitled* (1989), Bill T. Jones, who choreographed and performed the work, recovers memories of his late partner, the dancer and choreographer Arnie Zane through a richly evocative mix of text, movement, and image .[28] This is the "photomontage" that Benjamin alludes to and its "revolutionary" power. In *Untitled*, we see Jones stripped to the waist, sweating from the effort of his dancing, eyes locked on ours, speaking through us to his dead lover. Early in the piece, Zane appears superimposed in the upper right corner of the screen, a ghostlike presence. We see him moving, and we hear his voice recounting a dream in which he imagines a workman with his shirt off and the home he shared with Jones. Jones speaks about places they visited together, people they knew, the time in the attic drinking spring water with Jones's mother, when she said, "You take care of my boy now, he ain't got no education." In *Untitled*, Jones's memory of his life with Zane is both recovered and inscribed simultaneously. *Untitled* recorporealizes Zane via the digital image montaged into the still-living inscription of Jones. In video, they are equally alive, equally corporeal.

In Richard Schechner's *Performance Theory*, the author describes a situation he calls, the "efficacy-entertainment braid." He speaks about a kind of performance that is designed to be efficacious—that is to effect transformation: "[N]o performance is pure efficacy or pure entertainment. The matter is complicated because one can look at specific performances from several vantages; changing perspectives changes classification."[29] In Jones's *Untitled*, the work is *both* efficacious and entertaining. Its efficacy lies in the recuperation of the specter of AIDS and homophobia, in the re-animation of Arnie Zane as a ghostly presence that reminds us of our own corporeality. The entertainment value lies in Jones's passionate movement, his voice, and in the artistry of the direction and cinematography. The screendance that seeks only to preserve the "integrity" of a piece of choreography via film or video may be efficacious in that it serves to archive the dance in its complete theatrical form and serves the choreographer as a specific communication tool. It may even be entertaining as we see in the example of televisual dance such as "Dance in America." However, it is not efficacious in advancing our understanding of the *form* of screendance; thus, there is no transformation in that regard. Schechner maintains that to effect transformation is to be efficacious. Efficacy both transforms and advances the art form.

In the process of efficacious art making, one may or may not create an entertaining work, though to follow Schechner's logic, efficacy and entertainment are always linked. To recognize the entertainment value of an efficacious work requires that an audience engage in the critical and analytical dialog. A screendance that is effective in broadening the boundaries of the form may not at first viewing seem like what we know to be dance. But the recorporealized body persists in recuperating the screen memory *of dance* at the intersection of moving bodies and moving pictures.

CHAPTER 4

The Advent of Video Culture

The cultural transformation brought about by the evolution of video technologies must be understood as central to any theory of screendance. This chapter, aims to provide a more thorough history of the early days of video art in order to contextualize its linkages to screendance; it makes a case for the way in which ideas about the body and its numerous performance tropes have moved laterally across all of the arts in the era of video culture. Video art came of age during a time when media in general was increasingly permeating every aspect of daily life. I consider here the influence of mediatized culture on dance and the arts in general and address the interrelation of media and the arts (including video art) in the 1960s and 1970s, which significantly altered the way the body was represented on stage and screen, so that video began to be associated with both liveness and performance.[1] As it relates to screendance, *mediatization* refers to the way in which dance is transcribed from its state of liveness to a kind of objecthood as a product of mass media technologies.

Before video was embraced by the art world, the cultural phenomenon of television captured the attention of the public and became ubiquitous in a relatively short time span after its invention. Pioneered in the 1920s and 1930s, television increased in popularity after World War II and, in its earliest incarnation, all television was broadcast live. Liveness made television subject to the same sense of urgency that one finds in theater: the sense that the event is happening in real time and, as such, the possibility of either failure or transcendence is imminent. Through the 1950s television's artistic possibilities were briefly explored in the United States by artists such as Ernie Kovacs, who "was one of the first entertainers to understand and utilize the television as a true 'medium,' capable of being conceived and applied in a variety of ways." Kovacs, in his regularly broadcast shows, "recognized the potential of live electronic visual technology and manipulated its peculiar qualities to become a master of the sight gag."[2] While Kovacs explored television at one end of the spectrum, live theatrical productions and anthology dramas such as *Playhouse 90*, which relied on the use of recently developed video technologies, explored another theatrical and dramatic approach.

As production costs rose and sponsorship exerted more and more creative control over writers and directors, such artistic experimentation gave way to news and entertainment. In 1960 the first-ever televised presidential debates between John F. Kennedy and Richard Nixon demonstrated television's ability to powerfully alter the landscape of mass culture. As the 1960s progressed, televisual images such as the Beatles' debut on *The Ed Sullivan Show* and Neil Armstrong's walk on the moon reached millions of viewers and embedded themselves into the American collective unconscious in unprecedented ways.[3]

Yet, most crucial for this book's interest in corporeal images is the television coverage of the Vietnam War, often referred to as "the living-room war" because it was the first war to be regularly covered by the nightly broadcast news: it was literally in America's living rooms thanks to the technology of television.[4] The startling images of the war that pervaded 1960s and early '70s culture forever altered the way in which the body was imagined and staged. Wounded soldiers, their bodies and psyches fragmented from battle, flooded our cultural consciousness. Broken and eviscerated bodies became the "others" by which we examined ourselves, the "whole" ones.

Mediated images of war—televisual bodies—though powerful in their context, were at the time generally viewed on smaller-than-life black-and-white screens. Thus, Michael J. Arlen notes that television may have made such images *less* "'real'—diminished in part, by the physical size of the television screen, which for all the industry's advances, still shows one a picture of men three inches tall shooting at other men three inches tall, and trivialized, or at least tamed by the cozy alarums of the household."[5]

As the bodies of returning soldiers became reintegrated into the public consciousness both in the flesh and via televisual imagery, they inscribed onto the culture a new and different sense of corporeality. The generation of artists who came of age during and shortly after the war in Vietnam was constantly confronted by these bodies and their mediated images. Unlike the aftermath of other wars, television made these images ubiquitous, and this manifested itself as a sense of absence and loss in the work of many visual artists, including Robert Rauschenberg and Bruce Nauman. As early as 1966, Nauman created works in numerous mediums that tracked the absence of the body and its performative capacity by creating casts out of plaster or epoxy resin. Nauman's cast sculptures were topographies of negative, residual space: the body's absence implied its presence, its humanity, and its corporeality. Mapping the body's absence in works like *Space Under My Hand When I Write My Name* and *Templates of the Left Half of My Body at 10″ Intervals*, Nauman framed the body as a landscape fraught with meaning ◑.

Indeed, a great deal of art-making practice in the 1960s reframed the body via its relationship to landscape, to the point of considering the body *as* landscape, a landscape in which the body became a "site": a site of battle, a site of discourse, and a site of negotiation. Through the camera's eye, the body mimicked America's vast western landscape with which the "earth-works" artists would soon become enthralled. Thus, one facet of the art world found a fascination with the body as the site of art practice (performance), and another found an equal fascination in siting works of art within the landscape (earthworks).[6] These two practices began to overlap in the work of dance filmmakers of the time, especially in work by Amy Greenfield and Hilary Harris, in which the body is seen both *as* a landscape and *of* a landscape.

This phenomenon is particularly evident in Greenfield's film *Element* (1973); here, Greenfield's naked body rises and falls from a sea of black mud until the body and the landscape are inseparable. Or, to look at another

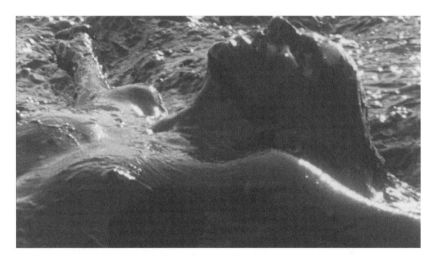

Figure 4.2: *Element* (1973), film still, Amy Greenfield
Photo courtesy of Amy Greenfield

example, Greenfield's *Transport* (1971) in which bodies—nonresponsive, limp as if wounded, in a sense "performing" death—are literally transported over harsh terrain. The other active and able-bodied performers carry and rescue the wounded ones while the handheld camera provides a shifting point of view, oscillating between first and third person.[7] Raised above the group as if on display, bodies fly through the air as if launched by canon fire. It is an image that speaks both of trust and of the necessity of saving or preserving the dignity of the damaged ones.

The iconography in this work, as well as in Greenfield's *Element*, represents a foregrounding of content enabled by quotidian formal elements. As such, these cine-dance works extend ideas from the Judson Church Group and also from Yvonne Rainer's prescriptions against virtuosity.[8] Though shot in film, they are relevant here for their destruction of linearity and the way in which the camera becomes a part of the *community* of performers on screen. The bodies in Greenfield's work cannot be read as *any* bodies; they are specific and recognizable as bodies of an era politicized by war—bodies in crisis.

Further fusion of the body and the landscape occurred throughout the 1960s, in work across multiple mediums as exemplified by the Italian artist Piero Manzoni, who stated that his actions were "the affirmation of the body itself as a valid art material" or Allan Kaprow, the American inventor of Happenings, who emphasized the body as the locus of artistic practice.[9] These artists were part of a movement that situated the work of art, or the locus of the work of art, within the body itself. It is interesting to note that the American choreographer Anna Halprin, whose own work was deeply influenced by Kaprow's, was a sort of hinge between the art and dance worlds. Halprin adopted numerous strategies in her community-based work that valorized and foregrounded individualism and the dignity of the body as a site of ideology, healing, and power. Halprin's *Parades and Changes*, first performed in 1965 and again in New York in 1967, provoked outrage by its use of matter-of-fact nudity as she tested the conventions of dance, social graces, sexuality, and authorship.

As these examples demonstrate, the body was central to many of the protean art practices of the 1960s, some of which left visible traces while others did not. In his series of performative *Body Prints*, the artist Yves Klein used the body both as tool and as mark, rolling bodies in pigment and then across canvasses to create "paintings" as a precursor to the ultimate negation of the act of painting. Klein's "paintings were now invisible"; the model had become "the effective atmosphere of the flesh itself."[10] Klein had already become well known for his 1960 work *Leap into the Void*, a single-frame photograph that depicts the artist frozen in midair, having leapt from the side of a building. While the authenticity and aftermath of this work has been questioned, it is emblematic of Klein's ideas about the ephemerality of the body. As with his *Body Prints*, *Leap into the Void* was the *reference* of a performative action.

Klein's "effective atmosphere of the flesh itself" manifested itself in the work of other artists as well. The Austrian artist Herman Nitsch created cathartic, bloody, and corporeal performances at his radical Orgien Mysterien Theater, beginning in 1957. These ritualistic performance actions, which often included music and dance, focused on the body as the site of ritual, staged crucifixions, and animal slaughter, thereby exploring the metaphors of life and death. They were pivotal, controversial works that involved all of the senses and used the body as their site of transgression. Further, they cleared the path for later 1970s performance art, which also explored the metaphor of the body. The German artist Joseph Beuys, for example, made the body (often his own) the site of discourse in works that emphasized the absence of a body, and in performances that blended ritualized movement and sound with materials such as honey, fat, earth, felt, blood, and dead animals. In works including *I Like America and America Likes Me* (1974), in which he lived in a gallery in New York with a coyote, and *How To Explain Pictures to a Dead Hare* (1965), in which, head covered in gold leaf and honey, he sat silently explaining pictures to a dead hare, Beuys embodied the object of art and its performative properties, as well as dematerialized the "thingness" of the work of art itself.

The artist Chris Burden took his version of body art to even greater extremes in the early 1970s with pieces like *Shoot* (1971), in which he instructed a friend to shoot him with a rifle, and *747* (1973), in which Burden shot a handgun at a jet passing overhead. These pieces reinforce the body as material for art practice, and in *Shoot* especially, the artist faces a very real risk of complete corporeal effacement. The art historian Henry Sayre says, "*Shoot* seems to elevate its artist/victim to the level of that elite group 'worthy' of the assassins bullet."[11] It follows that if the work of art is the body itself, then the value historically inherent in objects of art also necessarily shifts to the site of the body; thus Sayre's statement that Burden's body is "'worthy' of the assassin's bullet" underscores the cultural capital of performing bodies in the context of art practice.

Around the same time as Burden's early work, Eleanor Antin (see chap. 3) undertook a piece called *Carving, A Traditional Sculpture*, which she performed from July 15, 1972, to August 21, 1972. The artist's body was photographed on each of the forty-five days, during which time Antin followed a strict diet. As her body changed and ultimately became smaller (effacing itself in the process of becoming), she moved toward a culturally conditioned ideal of the body. Yet, Antin understood how that which is absent informs what is present, and how that which has been edited or effaced is that which must be banished in order to realize the ideal version of the body. Indeed, we will ultimately see that the notion of "editing" the body's presence is one that resonates laterally into the lexicon of screendance in an electronic environment as dance artists began to reconfigure ideas about choreography in the space of video.

The context out of which video and dance *merge* was thus highly influenced not only by the notion of the body as a site of performance but also as a movement away from the confines of traditional exhibition spaces. From the middle 1960s through the early '70s, visual artists began moving away from the paradigm of the gallery and the museum, and toward the landscape, a shift that resulted in the "earthwork" or "land art" movement. More broadly, this shift decentralized art practices and dislocated art products.[12] Artists such as Michael Heizer, Walter Di Maria, and Nancy Holt began siting work in the landscapes of the American West, creating viewing experiences that were predicated on the participation of the viewer. Robert Smithson's *Spiral Jetty* (1970), Di Maria's *Lightning Field* (1977), and Heizer's *Effigy Tumuli* (1983–85) were large-scale, ephemeral, site-specific work in remote landscapes, far from the art world both figuratively and literally. One was forced to trek out to them in order to see them, and even then there was no guarantee that they would "function" properly. Furthermore, as the work was often located in difficult terrain, viewing it required a type of physical exertion that was much more demanding than the typical art-viewing experience. The viewer thus became part of the performance in order to engage the work, a kinesthetic undertaking that literally enlivened the viewer's body.

Taking the work out of galleries and museums was an implicitly political action and rendered the work part of a much larger discourse about agency, presentation, and the nature of site as context. By moving away from the gallery system, the work became mythical in its absence. As the work outgrew the built environment, it also began to dwarf the bodies that managed to view it in person. The sheer size of these works called attention to their relative relationship to the body, their scale marking the body as significant, if only as a measuring device. Indeed, photographic documentation of earthworks—the way in which they were most often conveyed to the public—frequently features tiny figures in the foreground that convey a sense of the presence and scale: thus the body reinforces the heroic nature of the work. Earthworks so dwarfed human scale that they literalized the divine, transcendent experience that was the dream of pure, high modernism. And in this miniaturization of the corpus of the art viewer, it also made one acutely aware of the scale of the body in relation to the landscape.

Moving laterally across genres and mediums, we simultaneously find artists working with movement also situating their work in a dual site: within the frame of the camera and within a specific landscape in the natural world, outside of the confines of the theater. We see this in the work of Amy Greenfield and also in films and videos by numerous dance artists of the era including Carolyn Brown (*Dune Dance,* 1978) and Meredith Monk (*Quarry,* 1976).[13] The way in which Brown and Monk sited bodies in motion within a natural landscape amplified the possibilities of layered meaning in much the same way as visual artists working in the natural landscape. At the same time, siting the work within the specificity of film or video allowed dance artists to create work that was both portable and imminently replayable. It also allowed for the recorporealization of dancing bodies into a hybrid of site, corporeality, and media. This became the protean and malleable space of screendance.

The prevailing boundaries in mainstream film have, for the most part, kept dance artists from participating in filmmaking on a grand scale (with some exceptions, usually requiring collaboration and considerable funding), but these same boundaries have also created a rich history of so-called underground or experimental filmmaking. Experimental film, though materially and historically distinct from video art, laid a foundation for video culture and was a precursor to the use of media as an extension of visual art practice (video art). In addition, where experimental film originated in the modern era (flowing from traditional or mainstream filmmaking), video (and the art that is predicated on its technologies, including digital media) is a product of postmodern culture. It is fractured, atemporal, ubiquitous, and extends and expands film's appetite for movement, voraciously consuming every aspect of popular culture and returning it to the consumer as a twenty-four-hour digital feed. There has been an enormous bleed of the avant-garde into popular culture, a phenomenon that has helped to lead to the demise of the avant-garde as such. Video art, once the purview of artists alone, has morphed into a populist methodology for socialization, communication, entertainment, and any number of undertakings that, while distantly related to the earliest days of video art practice, bears little resemblance to the rigorous nature of the actual projects made by artists in its nascent days. Additionally it is further morphing into "digital" culture. However, video art is a part of a distinct postwar trajectory, one that overlaps with that of the expanded definitions of both dance and the visual arts in the twenty-first century.

Indeed, artists working across all media types have historically sought new and alternative methods for reconceiving traditional materials. And often, while doing so, artists rethink and redraw the boundaries that separate discrete practices as well, so that relationships between disparate media move laterally across genres and resonate in multiple worlds. As an example, Jackson Pollock's now famous abstract expressionist paintings shocked some viewers and critics of the 1940s and '50s who were used to a canvas that had a center, a reference point, and a sense of symmetry and balance. Pollack's "drip paintings" decentered the canvas, resulting in a nonhierarchical space in which the paint and the gesture that created the looping, intersecting whorls of color offered a new vision of what painting—and the *act* of painting—could be. At the same time the choreographer Merce Cunningham was experimenting with a similar use of stage space in dance. Though materially distinct, Cunningham's egalitarian use of movement across a stage, in which the center was always shifting, echoed Pollack's expressionistic canvases. Pollack's and Cunningham's works share the expressivity of the gesture even without a linear narrative and without natural or realistic forms present in their respective spaces.

This mirroring across formal boundaries, which has impacted dance via media of all kinds, from drawing to motion capture, also reflects the oscillation between discrete art practices, which in turn has engendered paradigmatic shifts across and beyond those practices. As such, mass media has always had a shaping effect on the other arts. Indeed, traditional modern dance was born in the age of cinema, and its rhythms, narratives, and methodologies often mimic those of cinematic practice. Postmodern dance, meanwhile, is of the age of video. Its deconstructed form, quick changes of focus, and discursive references mimic the nature of, and properties of, the video medium. Intertextuality and polyvocality are hallmarks of postmodern practices, and we can identify instances in contemporary dance where the practice of contemporary media is formally quoted, and the metaphors of both modern and postmodern art are also signified.[14] For example, the work of the German choreographer Pina Bausch is often cited as "cinematic" for its use of "montage, cross fades, and fade outs."[15] But the confines of "cinema" as a referent for Bausch's stage work are too narrow, as Bausch's work also has deep and important references to theories of postmodern pastiche and appropriation. Bausch created dances whose expressionistic use of theater space draws the viewer into a world that might equally be described as painterly; much like a Jackson Pollack canvas, her work for the stage eschews a central reference point and refuses a linear narrative. Her work incorporates gestural movement that is far removed from any sort of "natural" state of physicality, as bits of text are spoken in seemingly random order, and choreographic continuity, beyond isolated movement tableaus, is difficult to read.

While Bausch's stage work is generally not directly mediated by technology, it is the scale of her work that suggests the cinematic, though that argument is predicated on the viewer's active participation as a kind of virtual editor.[16] Bausch's expressionist dance theater requires the viewer to actively participate: focusing, editing, and constantly creating context for what unfolds within the work. This is a kind of work that is emblematic of dance in the age of media; its dismantled and pastiched form is predicated on postmodern media practices of both authoring and reception. Scholars such as Erin Brannigan have positioned Bausch as a "cinematic" or "filmic" choreographer,[17] but perhaps Bausch's use of the sort of editing and composition techniques usually found on screens, while *shared* by film, have more in common with the nonlinear and alogical techniques of sequencing historically found in works of video art and other media. What is sometimes referred to as "cinematic" in regard to Bausch's use of gesture, fashion, and general performative attitude, flows more specifically from theater and even to some extent the "frozen gestures" found in advertising—both print and otherwise. Bausch's own description of her work as "dance theater" or "*tanzteater*," is a designation that acknowledges the *theatricality* of her highly gestural performance language. Montage, cross-fades, and fade-outs are techniques shared by all moving image technologies and are found in equal measure in television, animation, movies, and video art. As such, they do not belong to the cinema any more than another media.[18]

Bausch's work, I believe, is part of the larger discourse of performance. The nexus between Bausch and the history of *performance art*, though perhaps under-acknowledged in the dance world, has been consistently noted by interdisciplinary scholars and critics in other fields. Echoing the work of Rose Lee Goldberg and Richard Schechner, the authors of *Social Performance: Symbolic Action, Cultural Pragmatics, and Ritual* make the following observation:

> "Performance art" is a collective term covering a range of artistic activities and movements, that from the 1960s onwards, appeared in different domains such as the visual arts, (Joseph Beuys, . . . Rebecca Horn . . . Bruce Nauman . . . dance (Pina Bausch), theater (Robert Wilson) . . . music . . . and pop culture. . . . Most performance art resists the attempt at neat classification by references to traditional branches of art and turns this crossing and fusing of boundaries into a distinctive feature.[19]

The claim of the authors for performance art as an *art of resistance*, while not negating the possible resonance of historic models including film, reiterates the space of performance art as one that is inherently at odds with "traditional branches of art," which extends to historical models of cinema. Instead, performance art has consistently noted its own allegiance to and rootedness in *movements* as opposed to *disciplines*. Futurism, Dada, and Surrealism, all manifesto-driven movements of the early twentieth century, coalesced around conceptual frameworks embracing, in part, a type of anarchic understanding of art. Performance art, inclusive of such artists such as Pina Bausch, is in the continuum of such intentionality. Bernhard Giesen suggests:

> Performance art aims at the *destruction* of conventional narratives, genres, and structures of meaning to open up a space for new and surprising, frequently provocative and even deliberately absurd happenings. . . . In this respect performance art continues the tradition-smashing heritage of *modernism* and, in particular, of futurism. . . . In particular, in its postmodern version it relies more on irony and parody than on direct destruction.[20]

Bausch's work in its transition or migration to the screen retains its inherent nature, which seems to fit quite well into the description above. Her reliance on what has been called "the cinematic" or "filmic" is undertaken with similar irony and historical referencing, which can be found in most explications of performance art. Additionally, film has been appropriated by artists interested in undermining artistic conventions since its birth, as in the work of such artist/filmmakers as Rene Clair (*Entr'acte*) and Man Ray (*Le Retour à la Raison*). Bausch's "provocative" and often "absurd" work for the theater appropriates the conceptual framing of early twentieth-century movements as much if not more than those of "the cinema," as does art made in the era of video culture in the general sense.

Film culture exerts a significant presence across genres and practices, often resulting in slippages in the terminologies used to describe mediated dance made in the era of video culture. Such slippages result in misreadings of work and blur the boundaries of subsequent discourse prompted by them.[21] This may be (partially) due to the fact that many artists who came to video in its early stages were trained in other media, including film. The pioneering video artist, Woody Vasulka, who worked extensively with the choreographer Daniel Nagrin, noted:

> Our context was not really artistic when we started to work with video. It was very far from what I would recognize as art. . . . I was educated in film at a film

school. I was exposed to all the narrative structures of film, but they weren't real to me and I couldn't understand what independent film was. I was totally locked into this inability to cope with the medium I was trained in. So for me, video represented being able to disregard all that and find new material which had no esthetic content or context.[22]

Video was as much a material for art making as a forum or platform for *thinking about* art. The artist Vito Acconci has referred to "Video as an idea, as a working method, rather than a specific medium."[23] In all its indeterminacy, video, at least as an idea or a theory, has ultimately become the site of dance's postmodern exploration of self through the digital era, in most cases supplanting film as the medium of choice. This is generally due to the cost or the availability of film but also for esthetic reasons that have little to do with pragmatics and more to do with surface quality. As artists have explored video as a site of performance (screen performance), so too have dancers and choreographers sited their work within "video space."[24] Aided by the ever-diminishing cost of video production, "video dance" has become perhaps the most populated subgenre of screendance. As video technology became more transparent and user-friendly, many choreographers infiltrated the medium, often moving from film to video with great fluidity. Conversely, the fertile period at the birth of portable video technology was one in which many artists trained in other genres (including film and the visual arts), such as Ed Emshwiller, Elliot Caplan, Charles Atlas, and Nam June Paik, created lasting relationships with dance. This is a legacy that informs the contemporary practice of screendance.

Paik, generally referred to as the "father of video art," was a Korean video artist who, in the early 1960s, began making works that questioned the very function of television and its cultural capital in the West. Paik reordered the viewer's relationship to the television itself and also to the methods of transmission/reception to which we had become accustomed by using actual televisions to create sculptural works. In 1965 Paik created *Magnet TV*, in which he placed a large magnet on top of a seventeen-inch black-and-white television, thus interrupting and disabling the image. Edith Decker-Phillips explains the interaction between magnet and television set:

The magnet's force of attraction hindered the cathode rays from filling the screen's rectangular surface. This pushed the field of horizontal lines upward thus creating baffling forms within the magnet's gravitational field. If the magnet maintained its position, the picture remained stabile—apart from minimal changes caused by fluctuations in the flow of electricity. Moving the magnet caused endless variations on the forms.[25]

The net result of this intervention on Paik's part was that the image on screen was reduced to purely electronic movement, a kind of movement completely free of narrative, often lyrical and electronically improvisational. Paik undertook these kinesthetic experiments in the pre-digital age, when analog electronics responded directly to outside stimulus or external conditions, which could be used to make the reception intermittent and compromised. Creating "dance on screen" by altering the signal pattern of televisions was not Paik's stated intention, although this violation of the video signal later became part of the electronic toolbox of artists such as Shirley Clarke, who used image processing as an esthetic component of screendance. This early gesture by Paik can be seen as a metaphor for the mediated interaction between dance and its televisual image.

Paik's attention shifted from the architecture of television to the moving image itself when Sony introduced the first portable video system.

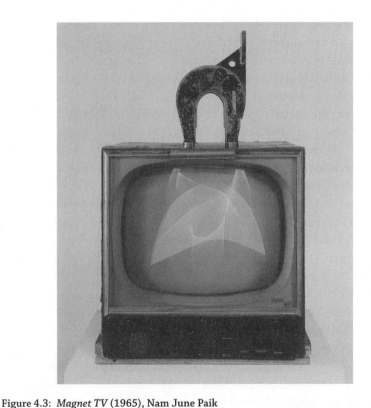

Figure 4.3: *Magnet TV* (1965), Nam June Paik
Nam June Paik, 1932–2006, *Magnet TV*, 1965. 17" black and white television set with magnet, 28 3/8 x 19 1/4 x 24 1/2 in. (72.07 x 48.9 x 62.23 cm).
Whitney Museum of American Art, New York; purchase, with funds from Dieter Rosenkranz 86.60a-b. © Nam June Paik Estate. Photograph by Robert E. Mates

In 1965 Paik was among the first to purchase one of these open-reel video decks and a black-and-white camera. As legend has it, after purchasing the equipment, on his way home camera in hand, his taxi became caught in a New York City traffic jam, caused by the visiting pope's motorcade. Paik pointed his camera out the taxi window and captured footage of the event, creating what many have cited as the first video art tape.[26] Later that same evening, he showed the tape at the Cafe au Go Go and handed out a leaflet proclaiming: "As collage technique replaced oil paint, the cathode-ray tube will replace the canvas."[27] In Paik's later work for television with Merce Cunningham, he continued to subvert and disrupt the image in a way that called attention to the materiality of the video signal, exposing or amplifying the hand of the artist.

Video art was therefore born of a moment when technology collided with a number of other phenomena, including the general path toward the amplified consciousness of the 1960s, as well as the promiscuous mingling of formerly autonomous art-making practices and the attempt to create space for new voices and methods within the art world establishment. In order to situate videodance (and screendance) within the larger culture of video art practice, it is important to excavate the relationship of performance *in general* to video *in particular*. Video began as a virtual tabula rasa in the art world; there were no rules and no historical tradition with which to conform in its earliest days. It was, in a sense, DNA-free. And since very few artists had production skills of any kind, video work could not be dismissed on the grounds of technical deficiencies. Virtuosity was neither expected nor required as an artist undertook the creation of a work of art in this new medium. Doug Hall and Sally Jo Feiffer, the editors of *Illuminating Video, an Essential Guide to Video Art*, note that such "anti-establishment beginnings" further distanced the makers of video from the experimental filmmakers that preceded them, while also distancing them from any other practice with a foothold in mainstream art culture. Hall and Feiffer contend that:

> Video's pedigree is anything but pure. Conceived from a promiscuous mix
> of disciplines in the great optimism of post–World War II culture, its stock of
> practitioners includes a jumble of musicians, poets, documentarians, sculptors,
> painters, dancers, and technology freaks. Its lineage can be traced to the dis-
> courses of art, science, linguistics, technology, mass media, and politics. Cutting
> across such diverse fields, early video displays a broad range of concerns, often
> linked by nothing more than the tools themselves. Nonetheless, the challenge
> of video's history has been taken on by the art world, though it might well
> have been claimed by social history or, for that matter, the history of science

and technology. Art historians, however, face two obstacles to constructing a credible history of video: video's multiple origins and its explicitly anti-establishment beginnings.[28]

Video practice thus came out of a milieu in which the very nature of art was under interrogation and in which media of all forms was both a key material for, and an integral tool of, its own circulation and dissemination, ultimately becoming a primary site of art practice. This site was both materially and intellectually separate from video in service of pure documentation of previously live events as the camera was seen to be an integral part in shaping such events. As a primary site of art practice, video's concerns and desires ranged from the corporeal to the political.

Moving from dance's abstract relationship to "the idea" of video and/or media to more concrete examples enables a closer focus on the historical relationship between video art and dance. Increased access to video technology from the 1970s through the 1980s made it possible for artists to consider dances for the camera as an alternative to theater dance (and also eventually impacted the way in which choreographers re-conceived the art of dance for the theater). In addition, it provided dance makers with a way to engage more directly with aspects of culture that dance could only tangentially address prior to its engagement with video art. Video allowed dance makers to think about both time and space, malleable constructs in the site of video, in a much different way than they might in live dance. Alternately, the ability for work in the medium of video to move about separate from its site of production, to be replayed on demand, was a way for dance to articulate its vision beyond the borders of its own history. Video annihilates time and space in a way quite different from film, with the possibility for instantaneous feedback and transmission, thus linking video dance practice *materially* to broadcast television media, which had become ubiquitous if not overwhelming.

The choreographer and dancer Daniel Nagrin, for example, who was featured in the work of filmmaker Shirley Clarke (*A Dance in the Sun*,1953) experimented extensively with video in projects with his New York–based *Workgroup* throughout the 1970s. Nagrin wrote extensively about the use of video in his own books as well and collaborated with the video artist Sholem Gorewitz on a number of projects, including *Steps* (1972) and *The Edge is Also a Circle* (1973). He was also featured prominently in the work of the video artist Woody Vasulka as the central character in Vasulka's 1988 landmark video work, *The Art of Memory*. Though both feature compelling performance by Nagrin, Clarke's *Dance in the Sun* and Vasulka's *Art of Memory* represent the polar ends of a spectrum of visuality in regard to the moving image. *Dance in the Sun*, a classic cine-dance of the period, begins in the dance studio and moves into the landscape (into "the sun") driven by Nagrin's dancing. It is reminiscent of Maya Deren's *Study in Choreography for Camera* in the way that the continuity of choreographic logic is carried between physical locations through the body of the dancer. *Dance in the Sun*, though fragmented by the editing of the "dance" inside its narrative structure, proceeds with choreographic integrity—the choreographic logic linear and unbroken from scene to scene, the film ultimately circling back on itself and ending the way it began, in the studio. In *The Art of Memory* however, Nagrin does not dance as such, but is rather a character embedded in the surface of a highly painterly and electronic landscape. *The Art of Memory* is densely layered and political, making use of the video-processing techniques that Vasulka engineered in order to attack and alter the surface of the video image, as well as to create metaphor and meaning from abstracted imagery.

In the San Francisco Bay Area, Skip Sweeney and Joanne Kelly of Video Free America (VFA), an artist-run media arts center that produced and facilitated video work by artists, were collaborating on such intermedia works as *Vidance* (1973) and performing their hybrid live dance/video intermedia works in San Francisco and New York. Their work attracted critical attention from its earliest stages. The dance critic Anna Kisselgoff, writing in the *New York Times* about a 1977 concert presented at the loft of Trisha Brown, described Kelly as "both a dancer-choreographer and a filmmaker" and noted the she combined video and live performance in order to minimize the separation of the two.[29] VFA also functioned as an exhibition space and laboratory for the work of Kelly, Sweeney, and others who were activists for hybridity and the merging of live and mediated performance. Partnerships, collaborations, and cooperative spaces such as VFA and the Experimental Intermedia Foundation, founded in New York in 1968 by Elaine Summers, were the fertile ground from which the overlaps between dance and video in the latter part of the twentieth century grew organically out of video's early "promiscuous mix" of practitioners.

The earliest days of the collaborative impulse between video artists and choreographers produced a number of screendance works that have become well known in the years since. Many of these were co-produced for television broadcast by such institutions as New York's public television station, WNET.[30] For example, *Blue Studio: Five Segments* (1975–76; part 1 of *Merce by Merce by Paik*), a collaboration between the video artist and filmmaker Charles Atlas and Merce Cunningham, was a virtual blueprint for a postmodern, fragmentary media practice that many artists have

adopted since its creation ❺. In dance circles, the work is most often attributed to Cunningham, while in the realm of video art, it is first recognized
as a work by Atlas. The piece is at least equal parts Cunningham and Atlas,
but its surface quality owes its provenance to video art and the image processing techniques of Nam June Paik (who collaborated on other parts of
the project). In *Blue Studio*, we see Cunningham in the studio, chroma-
keyed against a highway or road, occasionally joined by others, including
dancers, a dog, and his own mirrored image, in a two-dimensional electronic landscape. As the point of view and background constantly shifts
behind him, Cunningham "dances" with company members videotaped in
black and white in an earlier period of time, and ultimately his own electronic other. Taken as a gestalt, the collision of images with a score by John
Cage (which included snippets of conversation by Cage and Jasper Johns),
existing in a contingent electronic space, merges both form and content.
Blue Studio exemplifies a kind of nonlinear, pastiched, expressionist electronic space that would become a visual referent for a particular strand of
video art practice that valued the kind of image processing made possible
by early video technologies.

The importance of Cunningham's contribution to the development of
screendance is widely acknowledged, and his recognition of the camera as
a site for situating choreography, and the inherent differences between
camera space and theater space has led to numerous works for screen
along with a recognizable style of inscription. The resulting screen esthetic
is also largely due to the contributions of his collaborators—first Atlas, and
later Elliot Caplan, both of whom were media artists whose experimental
esthetics altered the visuality of dance as well. They and other many well-
known video artists, such as Paik, Mary Lucier, John Sanborn, and Skip
Sweeney, have crossed into dance for a time in order to collaborate with
choreographers in works that fused dance with video. Such collaborations
often push the envelope of contemporary dance by re-siting the choreographic impulse within a media landscape and within the specificities of
camera space. Conversely, the same collaborations modify and re-imagine
the space of video practice as bodies and their attendant histories are
foregrounded in electronic, digital, or synthetic space.

During its periodic forays into media space, dance has experienced
a transference of many of the particularities of media practice, and it has
absorbed much of the nature of media culture along the way. Dance, circulating in mass culture as it does, is highly susceptible to mediatization.
Contemporary choreographers such as Trisha Brown, Bill T. Jones,
Merce Cunningham, Anna Teresa de Keersmaeker, Bebe Miller, Susan
Marshall, and a host of others have been engaged with media in a range of

undertakings from documentary to screendance and media as part of a scenic design. They have all submitted their choreography to interpretation by film and video artists; numerous others, have invited media into their live theatrical dance productions in the form of projected images within a choreographic context. Such work has circulated widely among dance audiences, choreographers, students, and in academia as part of dance curriculums. Additionally, in the United States, Canada, Europe, and elsewhere, at least since the early 1980s, "dance for camera" has been seen regularly on television, if not in prime time, then at odd late-night broadcast moments. In fact, in the United States, broadcast images of modern dance go back to the live television of the 1950s.[31] It is safe to say, then, that choreography in both the modern and postmodern eras overlaps with media with some significance. Further, as choreographic works circulate among dancers and choreographers in digital or electronic form (on video, DVD, or the Internet), the way in which dance is created and ultimately consumed is altered by their mediated referent. When dance circulates via its mediated representation, it enters the domain of mass culture, or as philosopher Noël Carroll calls it, "mass art." Carroll refers to this mass art as a kind of distribution system that enables many people to perceive a work over and over in its mediated form.[32] Mass art, by its very nature, produces mass reception and the adoption of elements of those transmissions into art practices simply by exhausting resistance through repetition and frequency of delivery. But as Marshall McLuhan had previously pointed out, content is inseparable from form.[33] In other words, the content of every medium (in this case *dance*) is another medium (in this case *video* as the delivery system for the content of "dance"). And the content of both need also be considered for their individual and collective intertextuality, which helps to articulate or excavate meaning on a larger scale. While potentially fraught with meaning, mass art—works of art such as screendance made for mass distribution—must be systematically pried loose from the container of media in order to fully apprehend both the meaning and the value of such works.

Although screendance is decidedly a genre of contingencies, interrogating all of the parts of the whole (or system) may further illuminate the work. Hence the relevance of McLuhan's famous phrase, "the medium is the message," which indicates that "We can know the nature and characteristics of anything we conceive or create (medium) by virtue of the changes—often unnoticed and non-obvious changes—that they effect (message)." Furthermore, Mark Federman points out that, "McLuhan warns us that we are often distracted by the content of a medium (which, in almost all cases, is another distinct medium in itself). [McLuhan] writes, 'it is only too typical that the "content" of any medium blinds us to the character of the medium."'[34]

That said, screendance often overwhelms the viewer via the magic of the technologies by which it is produced, the stellar dancing or the lush landscape in which it occurs, to such an extent that it *resists* critique. This means that the delivery system of screendance, whether it be film or video or digital technologies, often becomes the only frame by which the work is cataloged or indexed, thus putting the work outside of a feedback loop typical to contemporary art in general. Again, in order to fully illuminate and critique both the form and its individual components, critique in *all* its manifestations must also be applicable to screendance in all of its manifestations.

Video is a technology but also a method of apprehension. Because we live in a digital age, video culture—the use of a camera (or simply a lens attached to a digital device) and instantaneous recording device—has instantiated a kind of looking that is embedded in all areas of our lives, including our art making. Video is a prosthetic system for seeing and materially affects the way in which we apprehend images, events, and other phenomena. Whether or not we actually make video ourselves, we are indeed a product of the video age, of video practice, of pastiche, and of cutting and pasting real-time video data as if it were simply text or words on a page. We embody video practice and in turn, we reinforce video practice as we *re*-make corporeality into art in the genre of screendance.

The incursion of media as a phenomenon, especially video, in the latter part of the twentieth century, clearly has consequences to both dance and the moving image. As McLuhan stated, "the personal and social consequences of any medium—that is, of any extension of ourselves—result from the new scale that is introduced into our affairs by each extension of ourselves, or by any new technology."[35] Any choreographer's interaction with media will necessarily result in not only an embodiment of media practices (if only by a kind of osmosis) but also an understanding of the content contained therein, as it is inexorably altered by the container in which it is delivered, i.e., *media*.

The omnipresence of media in the culture at large has been systematically mirrored in the dance world, and media has grafted itself onto the limbs of dance in both theory and practice to the extent that dance has become virtually mediatized. Symptomatic of media's infiltration into dance are not just those works transposed to the space of video (screendance, video dance) but also certain live choreographies that mimic the fast-paced cutting of television and film and that share space with projected images as semiotic shortcuts to an understanding of content. Such content includes place, time, narrativity, and choreographies that rely on normatives of beauty and entertainment which are often first introduced into the culture by television, film, and the new media.

Though there are many examples of this theory, the Bill T. Jones/Arnie Zane Company (see chap. 3) is a formidable live-dance company for whom media has become a part of their lexicon. In 1994 the company premiered a work for the theater titled *Still Here*. It was the culmination of a one-and-a-half-year process of reaching out to people with life-threatening illnesses through a series of "survival workshops" held across the United States. Though a "live" work, it employed pre-taped video to create a larger and more complex context. Working with the video artist Gretchen Bender, Jones was able to visually reference, on stage, the medical intervention into the body that comes with terminal disease and to bring into the theater the images of those with whom Jones worked during the creation process of *Still Here*. Using multiple projection screens, Gretchen Bender layered images of medical technology, the body and its organs, and the testimony of individuals cited in the text of *Still Here* to expand the architectural space of the theater into a multidimensional space, one capable of shifting into the past, moving throughout the body and speaking to us from prerecorded, subsequently silenced voices. By the use of projected video, the body is reclaimed as personal and expressive in a way that contextualizes the choreography of Jones on a level much deeper than a work performed on a bare stage. The images created by Bender allow for a sensual exploration of the diseased and disappeared body while providing a type of leitmotif or narrative against which we view the dance. The voices of the people Jones worked with across the country as he created *Still Here* come to us quite literally from the screen. The text spoken by the dancers from the stage references those seen onscreen, creating a dialog between mediated images and the present tense of the performance merging spoken language with video images into a hybrid language. Finally, the dancing is cast in a language that is clearly a language of the video age: fast transitions, jump cuts, a kind of *technique surfing* that mimics channel surfing in its relentless mutability, all sited within a frame of constantly changing and updating mediated information, coming to us (as often is the case in television) via talking heads. While not technically a screendance but rather a live dance performance with video (perhaps a *screenic* dance), *Still Here* is *video responsive* and specific to the desires of video culture. It is a grafted hybrid: responsive to and emblematic of video culture and a product of the migration of theory from other media-contingent practices in the age of postmodern mediatized culture.

In the years since that project, video culture has morphed into digital culture, and with that evolution, screendance has emerged as a locus of activity related to the technological mediation of performance. Within this hyperactive, even viral surge of production and exhibition, the discourse of screendance and screenic dance performance benefits from the neural network of its own provenance. Such a network is theorized here as an open architecture flowing from the visual arts, contemporary media culture, cinema, and dance practice as well.

CHAPTER 5

The Bride is Dance

In Marcel Duchamp's notes for his mixed media work, *The Bride Stripped Bare by Her Bachelors, Even (The Large Glass)*, the artist describes an erratic encounter between the "Bride," in the upper panel, and her nine "Bachelors," gathered timidly below in an abundance of mysterious mechanical apparatuses.[1] This delineation of gender and the objectification of the female (the object of desire) by her "bachelor suitors" is an apt metaphor for the marriage of dance and technology. Screendance, however, though clearly made possible by the marriage of dance and technology, sits on the periphery of, and is often absent from, that field's discourse. As the provenance of screendance can be traced to the birth of cinema (and further to the birth of photography), it is often considered to be part of the analog or "modern" histories; meanwhile, "dance and technology" tends to be viewed as of the twenty-first century digital world, thus placing it in a separate, "postmodern" discourse. This division is an artificial one: while the materiality of the technologies used to mediate dance has shifted considerably, what is constant is dance in relationship to technologies of representation as such. In other words, all technologies that mediate dance are of a piece, performing distinct roles, altering how we receive and perceive the performance of dance. "Dance and technology" seems a cumbersome term and is not entirely helpful in describing the actual practice, since it articulates the provenance of neither the dance nor the technology and implicitly maintains each term as separate and discrete. I substitute the term "mediated dance" instead, in an effort to merge dance *with* technologies of representation and to thus suggest a synthesis that avoids artificial bifurcation. Mediated dance then becomes an area of dance practice in

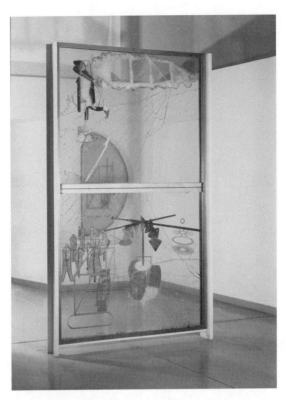

Figure 5.1: The Bride Stripped Bare by Her Bachelors, Even (The Large Glass)
(1915–23), Marcel Duchamp
Accession #1952-98-1
The Bride Stripped Bare by Her Bachelors, Even (The Large Glass)
Marcel Duchamp
Oil, varnish, lead foil, lead wire, and dust on two glass panels, 1915–23
9 feet 1 1/4 inches x 69 1/4 inches (277.5 x 175.9 cm)
Philadelphia Museum of Art: Bequest of Katherine S. Dreier, 1952
© 2010 Artists Rights Society (ARS), New York/ADAGP, Paris/Succession Marcel Duchamp

which dance is filtered through some element of media, whether camera-based, sensor-based, prerecorded, or otherwise intervened in via software or hardware, a technological interface or other device that modifies the dance in real or altered time. In this way, the subsequent discourse can become more specific to the technologies of mediation in a particular work or area of practice. And further, this sort of model necessarily includes screendance as a byproduct of such mediation.

As noted in chapters one and two, dance has been courted by techno-logically assisted image makers since the earliest days of photography and film. To extend the metaphor in Duchamp's *The Bride Stripped Bare by Her Bachelors, Even*, this courtship has resulted in numerous marriages between

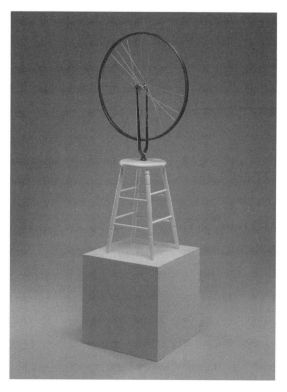

Figure 5.2: Bicycle Wheel (1913), Marcel Duchamp
Accession #1964-175-1 Bicycle Wheel Marcel Duchamp
Wheel, painted wood, 1964 (replica of 1913 original)
Diameter: 25 1/2inches (64.8cm)
Base height: 23 1/2 inches (59.7 cm)
Philadelphia Museum of Art: Gift of the Galleria Schwarz d'Arte, Milan, 1964
© 2010 Artists Rights Society (ARS), New York/ADAGP, Paris/Succession Marcel Duchamp

the Dionysian bride that is dance and her technological/rational bachelor suitors producing the contemporary offspring of mediated dance.[2]

For Duchamp, the object created by mechanical reproduction was an object full of artistic potential; it was simply in need of a frame of reference or *re*-contextualization. Both screendance practitioners and those engaged with other approaches to dance and technology are historically linked to the work of Duchamp; his concept of the "readymade" informed art-world ideas about technology and appropriation and helped to subvert entrenched ideas of authorship and the concept of "the original."

Duchamp used the term "readymade" to describe works of art he made from already manufactured objects. Choreography, once "set" might be thought of in a similar way. As choreography becomes codified and inscribed through repetition and performance, it becomes, in a sense, objectified and reproducable. In the process of mediating dance in camera space one of two strategies is often employed: choreography is created in the moment of inscription, or a preexisting choreographic work is remade in camera space. Collaborations in which dance is made simultaneously with its mediation may seem to fall outside of the Duchampian readymade paradigm—for instance, if the dancer improvises for the camera or other technological device (motion capture, etc). Yet (to again cite Sally Ann Ness's idea of the body as "host material" for the inscription of dance) improvised movement, even as it is being recalled in real time, is stored in the body as raw data, much like data is stored on a hard drive, and is immediately retrievable by the dancer. It is preexisting, living within the body, and mechanically reproducible into danced moments when demanded by the performer. It is readymade in relation to its mechanical reproduction and subsequent inscription in replayable media. Choreography, then, in relation to screendance, might be thought of as the readymade equivalent of Duchamp's off-the-shelf, pre-made objects of desire especially *if* the substance of the dance—the choreographic material—has been previously created, prior to its migration to media; and *if* the collaboration between the dance/technology partner and/or the screendance maker is after the fact of that creation.

Duchamp's ideas about the readymade extend to the edges of screendance, where it merges with contemporary art's ideas about appropriation as well. David Hinton and Yolande Snaith's *Birds* (2000), a screendance made entirely of found footage of the movement of various birds and then reedited to create a "dance film," is an example of both technological appropriation and Duchampian reframing. *Birds* mimics the gesture of appropriation found in many early experimental video art works by reframing and repurposing extant clips in ways that ask the viewer to reconsider the nature of the original material. In the ten-minute film, archival footage of birds in their natural habitat is cut together against a soundtrack of bird sounds and spare, rhythmic music. This kind of gesture is contextualized by both the venues that present the work, as well as the provenance of the makers of the work. Thus, the filmmakers—Hinton, a well-regarded director of screendance, and Snaith, an equally respected choreographer—remediate Duchamp's object-specific ideas about framing within a screendance context.[3]

The nexus between Duchamp and contemporary screendance can be found in work by other filmmakers including Shirley Clarke (see chap. 4). Best known for her work as part of the New York independent film community in the 1950s and 1960s, Clarke began her career as a dancer in the 1940s studying in New York with teachers including Hanya Holm. In Clarke's film *In Paris Parks* (1954), the director shot and gathered images of quotidian movement in various Parisian parks and edited it into a lyrical, rhythmic, short film. In *Bridges Go Round* (1958) Clarke creates movement pieces from stock footage of bridges and skylines shot in New York and again edited into a film that despite its lack of the physical presence of dancers has a distinct choreographic sensibility. *In Paris Parks* and *Bridges Go Round* are most often screened in the context of independent or avant-garde cinema as that community has contextualized much of Clarke's work. However, Clarke herself has claimed these works as cine-dance. As in the case of the Hinton films, though, both of these films rely on the contextualization of venue and curation to be considered in the larger discourse of screendance.

In their respective screen work, both Clarke and Hinton used readymade movement and reframed it via editing to pose questions about the nature of dance. Both adopt an approach to screen performance that flows from a similar impulse found in Duchamp's readymades and his ideas about appropriation and mechanical reproduction. And both suggest that "dance" is located not only in the performance of vernacular movement but also in the natural world and the built environment as well. Further, their work suggests that applying a particular frame to vernacular movement, dance is already there for the seeing: it is, in fact, readymade.

Flowing from the influence of Duchamp, the practice of appropriating one thing and framing or recontextualizing it as another has other antecedents and parallel histories as well, for example, the composer John Cage's well-known performance, 4′33″ created in 1952.[4] First performed by David Tudor, the pianist sits at the keyboard in silence (for exactly four minutes and thirty-three seconds) for three movements in which no notes are played, forcing the audience to simultaneously consider the nature of music and the "found" sounds of their surroundings as musical phenomena. This work by Cage repurposes Duchamp's ideas about the readymade and extends the conceptual frame to performance thus opening up the discourse to other media as well. Subsequently, and perhaps more directly related to the discourse of dance and technology, Cage presented a work called *Variations V* at Philharmonic Hall in New York in 1965. The piece was a collaboration with choreographer Merce Cunningham, musician David Tudor, and a host of artists, dancers and technologists in which the stage itself was fitted with photoelectric sensors by which the dancers movements triggered sound, video and lighting effects. While created in a decidedly analog environment, this model of interactivity is still prevalent today, though now migrated to the digital environment.

Variations V was a catalyst for a number of such experiments and during this time Cage, David Tudor, and a number of choreographers who had worked at the Judson Church in New York began to collaborate on events combining technology with performance. In 1966, the physicist Billy Klüver and Robert Rauschenberg collaborated on a project that brought together thirty engineers with artists to produce an event called, "Nine Evenings: Theater and Engineering." The engineers of "Nine Evenings" were not used to working within theatrical confines, and the artists were not used to the very precise, costly, and time-consuming nature of working with technology. Even though "Nine Evenings" has, over time, become highly influential for generations of hybrid artists. Furthermore, this inter-action was useful in beginning a dialog between artists and technicians, and in setting the stage for future interdisciplinary collaborations.

Rauschenberg continued his relationship with dance and technology through his collaborations with choreographer Trisha Brown, including the work *Astral Convertible* (1989), in which the dancers movement triggered sound and lights via onstage towers. *Astral Convertible* combines dance and technology without the usual hierarchy of disciplines, i.e., dance is not privileged over the scenic and interactive stage elements, but rather what is presented on stage is a synergistic hybrid. Trisha Brown's choreography maintains its integrity at the same time engaging the technology that Rauschenberg used in his stage design, and the piece functions as an integrated work of art.

Indeed, *Astral Convertible* occupies a territory that may be referred to as "the active stage." The active stage describes a kind of work that, while still bound to the theater, uses technology and/or media to suggest a shift in location, time, and context. Additionally, it supports a kind of relocation to a hybrid inside/outside space—a literal bringing of the outside in. Maya Deren's work in film used the camera to unbind the dancer from location (e.g., in *A Study for Choreography and Camera*, Talley Beatty moves cinemat-ically from one location to another). And thus we can see that cine and videodance has long relied on the suspension of actual time in deference to mediated time. In the inside/outside paradigm, the active stage replaces or augments static two- or three-dimensional object-oriented design with mediated imagery in the form of projected film, video, or digital data in order to create a permeable and mutable visual environment. Such an envi-ronment allows the author to layer visual signs of dislocation, taking the viewer literally outside of the theatrical space. This type of meta-dance has its roots in the work of the Futurist performances of the early 1900s and even earlier in Wagner's concept of *Gesamtkunstwerk*, or "total work of art,"

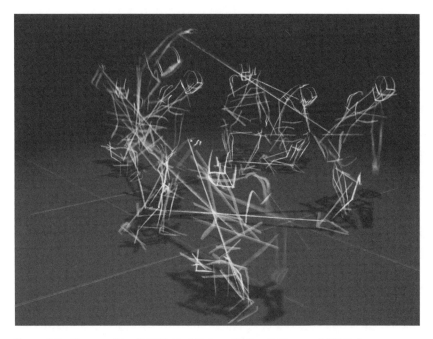

Figure 5.3: *Ghostcatching* (1999), Paul Kaiser, Shelley Eshkar, and Bill T. Jones
Still frame from Ghostcatching (1999) by Bill T. Jones, Paul Kaiser, and Shelley Eshkar, courtesy, the artists

in which the gestalt of multiple elements superseded each singular contribution.

We can locate the contemporary application of these ideas in the milieu of mediated dance, where the marriages between dance and technology are often ones in which the dancing bride is the articulator of the technologist's visual prosthetics. Those prosthetics may include cameras; motion-capture devices (as in the case of choreographer Bill T. Jones and Paul Kaiser/Shelley Eshkar's *Ghostcatching*); triggering devices (such as those designed by the Canadian media artist David Rokeby for *The Very Nervous System*; and interactive software like *Isadora*, created by Mark Coniglio of Troika Ranch (with choreographer Dawn Stoppiello). These are technologies that rely on dance (or movement): in many cases, the dancer may trigger a device that sets an event in motion, but the technology that enlivens the gesture is reliant on that gesture as an initiator. The dance therefore makes visible the technological device (and vice versa), and writes it in space (by triggering a sound or a media event, lighting change, etc.). Though the gap between the performed movement and the technological apprehension of it is minimal, time has passed, and it remains that

the technological suitor is appropriating the object of desire—the dance—
by reframing it and *re*-presenting it. This phenomenon was already
present in Duchamp's appropriation of readymade objects (although the
gap between production and apprehension was certainly longer); that
appropriation and subsequent exhibition in *art space* made the device
created by mechanical reproduction visible while writing the object into
a new context.

In the theory of the active stage, the site of the camera is also expanded
and returned to the stage to reinforce the choreographic vision by providing external source material as well as imaging a landscape, individual, or
place beyond the stage. Artists may employ projected images to quote
or cite phenomena located in other temporal or spatial environments or
to create a cinematic, narrative space in which to site choreographic ideas.
The epic *Still Here* (1995) by the Bill T. Jones/Arnie Zane Company is an
example of a theater dance work that employs video to create a larger and
more complex context within the active stage paradigm (see chap. 4).

There is another aspect to the active stage that relies less on moving
pictures and more on the transmission and re-casting of data into
animated spaces and objects via software and programming. Certainly, artists in the analog era undertook numerous experiments with motion-sensing devices, but entering the digital age the possibilities for interactivity
greatly expanded. In the early 1990s at the University of Arizona–Tempe,
John Mitchell and Robb Lovell developed *The Intelligent Stage*. It was an
amalgam of existing and new technology that, through the use of camera-
based sensing devices, could analyze movement within pre-defined areas.
The stage then was able to respond to a dancer's movements and react in
accordance with the design of the composer, choreographer, or director.
These responses could include changes in environmental elements such as
lighting, sound, and video, or they might actually affect the structure of the
environment itself. The flexibility of the *Intelligent Stage* allowed artists
to tailor its many elements: where sensors are located, what kind of
actions the sensors were sensitive to, and what responses occurred when
actions were recognized. For instance, a dancer's movement could trigger a
laser disc (precursor to DVDs and retrievable QuickTime movies) of video
images or a previously stored clip of dialog, or it could be programmed to
trigger a number of events simultaneously. Through residencies and
other methods, *The Intelligent Stage* thus allowed artists to create a new
generation of technologically based performance works. *The Intelligent
Stage* was at the forefront of technological innovation at a time when
there were no readily available, off-the-shelf software programs to
incorporate into a performance environment and was integral in defining

a technologically malleable space that helped to create a new lexicon of mediated performance.

Theatrical performance is still framed by the architectural space and historical contingencies of the stage itself. The stage, as it exists in repose, in the dark, uninhabited, is a seemingly neutral environment. Unengaged, it is a passive space. Without dancers (or other performers) to articulate its architecture and its boundaries, it is much like an abandoned house. It projects a certain function, but that function is largely an imagined one until it is engaged by its inhabitants. As we know in the postmodern era, however, virtually nothing is or can be neutral, especially a space as fraught with history as the modern stage in its capacity as a space for dance. "The stage" then, is always a conceptual space that contextualizes all that occurs within its architecture. "Conceptual" because each stage space has its own particularity—though, admittedly, the term "stage" itself conjures a formal space for performing that offers the commonalities of lights, possibly a curtain and proscenium arch, and seating for an audience located somewhere beyond the fourth wall.

There are numerous ways in which a performer may engage the stage. The most commonly encountered in a dance performance context is a paradigm in which "the work" or the choreographic performance is "dropped" into the space with little interaction with the particular architecture of the space beyond pragmatic considerations. Those considerations as to sight lines, lights, audio playback, and the like are generally simple modifications of how the work may have been previously performed or staged in another theater. In this case, the theater is a passive recipient of the work, providing a venue more than anything else. Perhaps this is a byproduct of the fact that most dance is created in studios (for various reasons) and subsequently brought into the site of performance only shortly before the performance is to take place. This is quite different than a dance performance that grows organically from within a space or site, immutably hinged to the specificity of the site.

The second model for engaging stage space is largely based on a kind of "visual metaphor," or cinematic praxis. It is an attempt to activate the stage space in such a way as to supersede its residual historical contexts and simultaneously create an architecturally specific site-within-a-site. This specific site engages the existing architecture of the theater only marginally and only in the most functional way, as a housing for an often alchemically transformed space. Certainly "pure dance" can transform a space and provide a transformative experience for the viewer. However, the active stage in this case is one in which space is materially transformed as well as virtually and metaphorically.

In this example, the physical space of the stage is made malleable by the use of technological interventions including telematics, prosthetic devices such as wearable computers, motion-capture technologies, and software programs such as MAX/MSP, Isadora, and others that allow for instantaneous on-site mixing of live and recorded video or sound. These technologies may also completely jettison the physical materiality of stage space by siting "dance" in web-based virtual environments or in the digital landscape. As the staging of danced events becomes more digital and less corporeal, the courtship of dance, the relationship between the bride and her bachelors, becomes more tenuous. When dance is used to create data for a secondary applications such as motion-capture or triggering devices, it distances the viewer from the actual physicality of movement. There is a qualitative difference between the "liveness" of dance in its traditional theatrical setting and dance in its mediated, screen contingent forms (which includes screendance), although the borders of dance and media are becoming increasingly porous. That is to say that dance is increasingly infiltrated by media practices whether they be materially evident on stage or simply stylistically referenced by the choreographic choices made within a live unmediated performance ⊜.[5]

The technologies of representation used to create an active stage include the technologies of dance itself, the techniques of performance, and the meaning that accrues from the body as viewed through and in the site-specificity of a mediated visual landscape. For example, in works by Troika Ranch (a performance group working at the intersection of dance and technology) such as *Loop Diver*, co-created by Dawn Stoppiello and Mark Coniglio, the audience simultaneously encounters projected video, interactive triggering of live and prerecorded "events," scenic design, and complicated sound design as well as live dancing bodies. In processing multiple media simultaneously, the audience perceives meaning from the gestalt of information. This phenomenon speaks to the audience's increasing ability to process multiple streams of visual and/or aural information at a time, a by-product of an increasingly mediated contemporary culture.

In *The Return of the Real*, Hal Foster proposes a theory in which he tracks a strand of the avant-garde from Duchamp to Warhol and focuses on a kind of art practice that is situated in social sites and the materiality of actual bodies.[6] He surmises that as artists move beyond the traditional art-making materials of the past to more conditional materials, art has returned to the locus of the personal, of the body and its spaces of habitation. Perhaps this is the phenomenon that is being played out by dance makers as they increasingly rely on media and projected images within a theatrical performance, to imply a kind of "real" social site or landscape. A by-product of the mediation of live performers in theatrical environments, however, is the potential for the *disappearance of the body* within the site of technologically mediated dance and/or performance.

If we think of the active stage in relation to Foster's "spaces of habitation," then the intersection of dance and technology in a theatrical environment creates a specific site. *All* dance is site specific; dance is always *in situ*. Everywhere that dance occurs is a place—a site—whether it be a theater or a landscape or the crook of a tree, and as such the site impresses upon the dance a kind of imprint that is more or less visible depending on the nature of that particular site. Technology may also be thought of as a site, and the imprint that flows from dance's interaction with technology depends not just on how deeply the dance is embedded within the site but also the degree to which the technology is foregrounded or imposed upon the dance. Concert dance in a theatrical environment at its most basic has a quotidian relationship with technology vis-à-vis the use of lighting and other common technological mediation. We can think of technology in degrees of transparency and/or opacity, though. The more transparent, the less we notice it; the more opaque, the more it imprints itself and alters our perception of dance and the bodies that perform it.

From Leonardo da Vinci's *Vitruvian Man*, which as early as 1490 attempted to fuse artistic and scientific objectives, through *Taylorism* in the late nineteenth century to the interactive dance and technology projects of the current era, the desire to extend the body through prosthetic devices designed to amplify and articulate movement has been a constant 🔊. The intersection of dance and the technologies of representation has conspired to offer the viewer a panoply of digitally mediated and altered experiences of the body in motion. From telematic performance to media-filled staging to dance made specifically for the camera, the body is in constant focus and is a site of consistent negotiation as well.[7] However, digital manipulation of corporeal presence, of liveness, leads to a particular kind of distancing that tends to *re*-render the humanness *of* live performance into various forms of data, either in a live or postperformance paradigm. It is ironic that as live performance becomes more engaged with technological mediation, it begins to encounter problems that documentation of live performance has previously encountered. The use of the "live camera" to provide real-time mediation of live performance by companies as diverse as Troika Ranch, The Builder's Association, Joe Goode, and others conflates documentation with liveness to the degree that the theories associated with each begin to merge and confound each other.

As an example, in "Presence in Absentia: Experiencing Performance as Documentation-Performance Art Focusing on the Human Body in the Early 1960s Through the 1970s," Amelia Jones describes writing about performance that she has only experienced through documentation and ephemera. She finds "that there is no possibility of an unmediated relationship to any kind of cultural product, including body art." She continues,

> Although I am respectful of the specificity of knowledges gained from participating in a live performance situation, I . . . argue that this specificity should not be privileged over the specificity of knowledges that develop in relation to the documentary traces of such an event.[8]

What if the "documentary traces" of a live event are created simultaneously to that event and are intended to be perceived within the same temporal envelope? What if the "documentary traces" are manifest in the form of video imagery that doubles the presence of the live body, confuses past and present through projections or digital data, and/or traces the body's presence in space and time via motion-sensing or other data-gathering devices? Jones further complicates these questions when she writes:

> The sequence of supplements initiated by the body art project—the body "itself," the spoken narrative, the video and other visuals within the piece, the video, film, photograph and text documenting it for posterity—announces the necessity of (quoting Derrida) "an infinite chain, ineluctably multiplying the supplementary that produce the sense of the very thing they defer: the mirage of the thing itself, of immediate presence, or originary perception. The play of substitution fills and marks a determined lack."[9]

In the case of work created for the active stage, which is a specific site where the "supplementary" and the "mirage of the thing itself" are woven together—often in an attempt to *amplify* presence—Jones suggests that the theatrical product is a conscious choice in which the artist intentionally combines the live with its mediated representation. The tools of mediation, previously used to manage the past, are now called upon to function in the present in a way that defers the lack often found in the documentary ephemera of live performance—while, yet, pushing the viewer even farther away from the corporeal itself.

This persistent tension between the live and the mediated is the overwhelming condition of digital culture. The possibility of sequential or successive iterations of a work of art that compound and multiply, or the singular reception of the live event and its attendant yet fragile aura of "originality" are but one dialectic among many. In the digital world all events are generative, and for better or worse, the notion of "the original" can often seem quaint or antiquated. Still, the question of "humanness" has attached itself to the discourse surrounding mediated performance since its earliest incarnations.

In his essay "Is There Love in the Telematic Embrace?" (1990), Roy Ascott attempted to attribute to electronic art the potential to embody love. Mindful of the schism between utopian and dystopian perspectives on technology and the future with respect to art, Ascott addressed a common concern among critics of electronic art: the fear that technology would overwhelm and dehumanize the arts, a last bastion of humanist values. If it could be shown that telematic art had the potential to embody love, then it would not be a paradox for art to be electronic and simultaneously serve humanist principles. Ascott's use of the term "love" and his concerns about "humanism" are seemingly at odds with the rhetoric of distance and scientific cool that are commonly applied to this area of practice. Work made in the milieu of the telematic is often not categorized as art per se but rather as *research*, (especially in academic settings) balancing it precariously on the razor's edge where science collides with the humanities.

Ascott proposes the following:

Telematic culture means, in short, that we do not think, see, or feel in isolation. Creativity is shared, authorship is distributed. Telematic culture amplifies the individual's capacity for creative thought and action, for more vivid and intense experience, for more informed perception, by enabling a participation in the production of global vision through networked interaction with other minds, other sensibilities, other sensing and thinking systems across the planet— thought circulating in the medium of data through a multiplicity of different cultural, geographical, social, and personal layers. . . . It is the computer that is at the heart of this circulation system, and, like the heart, it works best when it becomes invisible. The computer is the agent of the datafield, the constructor of dataspace.[10]

It is interesting to note the tensions in this paragraph. Ascott situates the "vivid and intense experience" of "creative thought and action" within the provenance of the mind and offers the metaphor of the computer as the "heart" of the circulatory system with agency over the spaces through which "data" circulates. The language that Ascott assumes begins to use the body as a trope for humanizing the computer, for assigning the computer's tasks to particular sites within the body. Meanwhile, the title of Ascott's essay immediately stakes out an important position that seems contradictory to the core of his theory. By using the term "telematic embrace," he suggests a very human gesture: technology wrapped around us in a way that might suggest compassion or nurturing. And yet the idea of technology as comfort-giver conjures a different set of images: it suggests coldness, hardness, and surfaces that distance us from our bodies.

It may be logical, then, to assume that the nurturing aspect of the telematic embrace be found not in the *form* of such work, not in its surfaces but in its *content*. It has long been the project of performance to speak in the first person, to instantiate content, and by extension *meaning*, into art practice through embodied actions. Yet we might also say that in media-based work found in the active stage, form often presumes content as an outcome of the juxtaposition of images on stage. As contemporary media practices migrate into live dance, meaning is increasingly contingent on the image set in which the dance is immersed.

The media theorist Lev Manovich goes a step farther in the body/mind/computer metaphor, and this allows us to connect the navigation of digital datafields to the way that we embody or map social and/or performative spaces:

> The very principle of hyperlinking, which forms the basis of interactive media, objectifies the process of association, often taken to be central to human thinking. Mental processes of reflection, problem solving, recall and association are externalized, equated with following a link, moving to a new page, choosing a new image, or a new scene. Before, we would look at an image and mentally follow our own private associations to other images. Now, interactive media asks us to click on a highlighted sentence to go to another sentence. In short, we are asked to follow pre-programmed, objectively existing associations.[11]

While Manovich is speaking specifically about new media, his point about "interactivity" may be applied equally to live performance in a mediated environment. Both Ascott and Manovich suggest a kind of embodiment of digital technology, one that is full of human metaphors but one in which it seems that we as participants/receivers/viewers are marginalized by the systems we seek to inhabit: creative systems with predetermined or overdetermined "maps" for navigation and a computer at the heart of the system. These are systems in which the real metaphors of the body, the alimentary, the decrepit, the erotic, and the undependable are curiously absent from the rhetoric. In short, they lack the very aspects of humanness that conspire to create events and experience that are elating, disappointing, frustrating, and moving—the very properties associated with liveness in theater, dance, and performance.

While artists tend to be early adopters of new technologies, media based art practices have often been cautiously approached by critics and theorists. In her essay, *Against Interpretation*, Susan Sontag, in speaking of Plato, notes that: "the earliest *theory* of art . . . proposed that art was mimesis, imitation of reality. . . . It is at this point that the peculiar question of the value of art arose. For the mimetic theory, by its very terms, challenges art to justify itself."[12] In the contemporary era, the avant-garde looked beyond the figurative, beyond mimesis, to a more subjective mode of representation and self-expression. However, Sontag states, "content still comes first . . . it is still assumed that a work of art is its content." She makes the claim that "the idea of content" is mainly a hindrance or nuisance, in fact, "a philistinism."[13] Sontag casts the desire for content and by extension, meaning, as a sort of lowbrow, blue-collar pursuit, one in which the viewer indulges her need to understand a work of art as opposed to simply embodying it, to interpret it rather than to experience it. The essay is at once compelling and irritating as Sontag makes her argument against interpretation or what she refers to as "the perennial, never consummated project of *interpretation*." She continues, "it is the habit of approaching works of art in order to *interpret* them, that sustains the fancy that there really is such a thing as the content of a work of art."[14]

Sontag's essay was written in 1964 during the height of Greenbergian modernism and its attendant form/content dialectic. What Sontag is focusing on is not *that* particular argument but rather the notion of the transformation of visual culture and myth by means of "scientific enlightenment." She speaks specifically about the discrepancies that arise as ancient texts are engaged by contemporary readers through interpretation, a process meant to disclose its "true meaning" by making the text "intelligible." In the translation of opaque or mysterious texts, therefore, the truth is liberated and enlightened for the lay reader. "The interpreter, without actually erasing or re-writing the text, *is* altering it [claiming] to be only making it intelligible, by disclosing its true meaning."[15] Sontag gives, as an example, the biblical story of the Exodus from Egypt and the Jews' wandering for forty years, finally entering the promised land. She notes that the story has been translated into an allegory of "the individual soul's emancipation, tribulations and final deliverance." She explains: "Interpretation presupposes a discrepancy between the clear meaning of the text and the demands of later readers [and] seeks to resolve that discrepancy." She further states that, "Interpretation is a radical strategy for conserving an old text which is thought too precious to repudiate by revamping it."[16] While Sontag builds her argument by using the example of sacred or religious texts, she also expands it outward to engage Freud and Marx's "elaborate system of hermeneutics" in which, "all observable phenomena are bracketed, in Freud's phrase, as manifest content."[17]

All events as well as texts are therefore to be probed for their "true meaning"; for Freud and Marx, Sontag suggests, there is no meaning without interpretation.

As in the interpretive process of Duchamp's *Large Glass*, however, which yields a theoretical premise, the intellectual reception of art does not necessarily negate the sensual reception of the same work. Ascott writes, "Meaning is the product of interaction between the observer and the system, the content of which is in a state of flux, of endless change and transformation."[18] Meaning, then, is neither fixed nor not-fixed, but flexible and porous. It is both a part of and apart from the attempt to interpret. By combining Sontag's and Ascott's theories about the reception of meaning, we come to a synthesis that requires not only the embodiment and physical pleasure of a work of art but also the subsequent intellectual encounter that further contextualizes the experiential nature of the work. This synthesis enables us to understand the juxtaposition of image and performance in works such as *The Light Room* (2002), by the Australian dance artist Hellen Sky, as constantly asking that we consider the relationship of the body to technological mediation and insisting that meaning is a fluid construction of all of the elements present in the active stage.

Mediated performance, telematic or otherwise, is cinematic in that it often asks that we suspend disbelief, to not interpret, but to allow

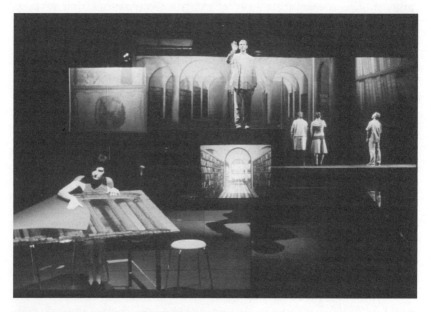

Figure 5.6: *The Light Room* (2002), **Hellen Sky**
Photo courtesy the artist

ourselves to be immersed in its technologically produced space. But to ignore the seams and overlaps, the grafted spaces of mediated performance, is sometimes difficult. So-called live processing or images projected within a "live" event are subject to a kind of digital lag or interpolation. And so the bodies we see on screen are not *our* bodies, nor are they "real bodies" in "real time" and the spaces they exist in are virtual or synthetic. Yet, the impetus to embrace their humanness, the desire for them to *be* human and to commune with them is palpable. Texting, e-mailing, motion-capture and telematic performance are all of a piece; relying on the imagined humanness of the mediated other, one that we either attempt to commune with directly or one that we voyeuristically desire from a safe distance. They all speak to a longing that extends beyond the functionality of technology.

Media-based practices including telematics, web-based, interactive and or digitally mediated performances are often perched in the liminal space between art and science, or between practice and research. It is in this liminal space that the courtship between the bride (dance) and her bachelors (technology) takes place. The recollection of Duchamp's readymades suggests that perhaps this courtship requires a *re*-framing that is an amalgamation of the cumulative theories of dance, new media, performance, and emerging technologies. Just as Duchamp's *Large Glass* is played within the active stage contained within its edges, yet pushes against them, so too does dance in the frame of mediated performance push against its own frame.

CHAPTER 6

Excavating Genres

Screendance is a diasporic culture, one that constantly migrates through host cultures and assumes various vernacular elements, while often struggling to maintain both its empirical elements and the identity of its "culture(s) of origin." At the core of this dynamic is this: the techniques of representing images on screen also flow from preexisting genres and so have material specificity that is readable as well. Both dance's and media's contingent origins thus conspire to create meaning that emerges from the cumulative effect of their grafting: traversing both temporal and physical geographies, dance and media absorb something of the landscape and culture of each, thereby generating communities of practice that share both common languages and stylistic elements. These "imagined communities" exist across international borders and are linked via a diasporic family tree that are readable through the cultural objects they create.[1] It seems accurate to claim, though, that if both disciplines that make up the whole of a screendance have traceable affiliations with genres, then we should also be able to name the resulting genre into which the new work falls. In other words, screendance may be thought of as the product of a lineage that can be articulated in various ways, including the provenance of the dance language within the work; the materiality and history of the media by which it is created; and also the complex cultural migration of its makers and its references.

As screendance in its institutionalized form—and more specifically in its nascent academic form—becomes historicized, and as that knowledge subsequently informs the practice, the field benefits from theoretical disruptions that question and disturb the received knowledge, replacing or

augmenting it with alternative modes of inquiry. In this chapter, I introduce a narrative of screendance that emphasizes distinctions between
genres, medium specificity, and identifiable difference flowing out of formal
or substantive approaches and concerns. By examining screendance alongside the structure of other art forms, the discourse around screendance
might be made stronger by excavating and identifying its generic sources,
which would in turn push screendance into a broader and more vital
interdisciplinary dialog.

The information needed to unpack and describe individual works of
screendance emerges from the terminology and language offered by its
makers and presenters. To fully realize generic difference and to construct
a narrative of related screendance communities and genres requires a closer
reading of the practice, as well as some knowledge of the intent of the
authors. In his book *On Criticism*, Noël Carroll points out:

> One very important access road to the intentions of artists has to do with the
> fact that artists produce works that belong to acknowledged categories. That is,
> in general, artworks belong to categories—like genres, styles, movements, peri-
> ods, oeuvres, etc.—and/or they have lineages and traditions. We can locate the
> pertinent kind or combination of kinds to which the artwork belongs by, among
> other ways, calculating the number and salience of features that the work being
> criticized has in common with members of the prospective class of artworks
> which we suspect it belongs.[2]

It is clear that by cataloging the relative attributes of artworks within a
greater context, we can derive further meaning and partake of a larger cultural dialog catalyzed by each work of art. Genres do not readily announce
themselves, though, and this is where the process of excavation must be
undertaken. While the quantitative methodology that Carroll cites is integral to the way in which the art world functions as an evolving intellectual
community, screendance has been resistant to most efforts to articulate its
genres and categories of practice, even given the thoughtful and considered
attempts to do so over the last decade.[3]

Manifesting this desire for a more rigorous viewing of the field, the
dance scholar Sherril Dodds published *Dance on Screen: Genres and Media
from Hollywood to Experimental Art* in 2001, in which she articulated a
number of screendance genres. Dodds quotes screendance makers and
directors who point out influences for their work that come from sources
outside the dance world. She notes, for instance, that the director "[David]
Hinton's fascination with the possibilities of movement on screen does not
derive from a dance tradition, but from popular action films."[4] In this case,

Hinton appears in a spectrum of artists whose work flows from very particular genres with equally particular esthetic and material concerns. It falls to those who consume and circulate the resulting work to further articulate the meaning of those concerns when they are attached to a particular dance vocabulary in a film or video hybrid.[5]

Dodds's book articulates theoretical paradigms that have gone largely unchallenged since its publication. In a recent essay "Does Screendance Need to Look Like Dance?" Claudia Kappenberg speaks back to Dodds, suggesting a number of alternatives to parsing the field into genres and noting that "a limited vocabulary for the discussion and critique of such work has continued to tie screendance practitioners and ambassadors to the pre-existing disciplines" that Dodds articulates.[6] It may be that the screendance community lacked sufficient critical mass to mount a response to Dodds's challenges for a higher degree of criticality; as the practice has grown in the last decade and as more exhibition venues have appeared, however, there has been a persistent resistance to adopting the same rigor found in the larger art world by which the community creates a vocabulary to articulate its process and practice.

That is not to say that genres are necessarily fixed: as dance is mediated within the site specificity of camera space and by the material cultures of film, video, or digital technologies, it tends to assume the characteristics of that mediation. In the diaspora of dance through the culture of media, dance tends toward film or video, while simultaneously attempting to maintain its autonomy (see fig. 6.1). At the top of the graph, dance is subject to a higher degree of mediation, in the form of cinema and/or television. At the bottom of the graph, dance—closer to its live performance—is subject to a lesser degree of mediation, which might be through documentation or postproduction. For example, if its migration is through the system of television, it *becomes televisual* as it assumes the characteristics and boundaries of the medium of television. Those specificities include duration, production values, and other recognizable characteristics of television. Dance tends to conform to the space of media, to its pace, to the patterns of viewership and distribution, and to the way in which media objects are consumed. Conversely, if the end point of a screendance is the cinema, it would be safe to expect that the makers of such a work might imbue it with a larger-than-life sense of scale and with the hallmarks of cinematic style and conventions, including framing and editing styles, narrative logic, and the like.

If we consider the way in which screendance is *spoken of* from a critical viewpoint, it is clear that the discursive language of dance tends to persist. This may be because the genre's normative viewership is most often within

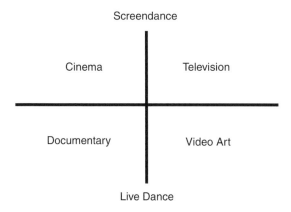

Figure 6.1: Axes graph, Douglas Rosenberg
© Douglas Rosenberg

the context of a dance audience. The way in which dance on film or screen-dance tends to be discussed and critiqued thus depends on the intellectual point of origin of the *speaker*. If dance and its diaspora are privileged by the speaker/viewer, the language of dance will be the currency by which the work is critiqued. If the speaker/viewer privileges film or video (and its diaspora), it is likely that the language of the moving image will lead the discourse away from issues of kinesthetic and/or choreographic observations.

Choreographers have actively extended ideas about site-specificity, engaging the screen as site for dance. However, it is always a site that is doubled: the initial layer is the built environment or landscape in which the body (dance) is located; the secondary layer is the media by which the performance is inscribed, bonded into one screenic image. In short, the visual culture of screen-based dance cannot be separated from the signifiers present within the frame itself and in the device by which that frame is created. Meaning flows from the entire image as well as its fragmented parts, often exposing the numerous tensions between the two and the competing desires of each.

On screen, dance seems simultaneously to resist and to adapt to the space of media—to its pace, to the patterns of viewership, and to the way in which media objects are consumed. One of the tensions that arises is the way in which the language used to describe the cohabitation of dance and media tends to also describe a service-based relationship. For instance, the often-used phrase, "dance for camera" (a common festival title)[7] implies that it is dance that is being staged at the *pleasure* of the camera, for the express purpose of the camera's desire.[8] It also implies that the camera is a spectator or receiver of the dancing body as opposed to a space in which dance flows with the agency of a collaborator. Thinking laterally, it would seem odd to use a phrase such as "acting for camera" to describe a similar hybrid, for instance a "narrative film," unless it be in the context of a course on the practice. Dance for camera does not imply a course but rather a course of action, a privileged performance made specifically for the viewership of the camera-eye.

The use of the word "for"—as opposed to "with" in this phrase is fraught with meaning. It implies a slavish relationship in which it is the camera *for which* all is performing, a hierarchical suppression of dance as a method of communication with its own agency and desire, and a casting of camera space as a kind of colonial space for which dance is simply another subjugated citizen. In this case, both dance and the camera ultimately suffer. These linguistic constructions tend to reinforce the difficulties in critiquing such hybrid forms, as they maintain a material binary by continually restating their cultural and material affiliations. Dance/camera, camera/dance: either way, such terminology allows for the viewer/consumer/critic/ theorist to attach their gaze on either solely dance or solely the camera, virtually piercing and eliding the hybridity of the form before their eyes. In order to think of screendance in more relative terms, this graph (fig. 6.2) defines a spectrum of signifiers.

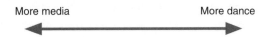

Figure 6.2: **Flow graph, Douglas Rosenberg**
© Douglas Rosenberg

Quite simply, the relative location on the graph where the screendance is placed speaks to the material nature of the work. Work residing on the "More Dance" side of the spectrum will, by nature, be more recognizable as dance. Here, media is a support device for the exposition of dance as a subject. If a work falls on the other end of the spectrum—"More Media"—it is likely that the work will be most identifiable as a work of media in which dance is merely a part of the overall composition and screenic quality of the work, objectifying it and claiming it as materiality. The exact center of the graph would therefore signify a hybrid of both media and dance, with each receiving equal consideration both artistically and conceptually. While this graph speaks to the relative proportionality of media and dance within a work, it is also concerned with how screendance might be more fully articulated in its hybrid form. If we consider screendance to be a subcategory of screen performance in general, then its tributaries might be envisioned as bubbling up from various extant genres including visual art, television, video art, dance, and so forth (Fig. 6.3). Subsequently, as new genres are identified as contributing to the culture of screendance, they too will frame such discourses surrounding the diasporic nature of screendance, its relationship with other media practices, and its general context.

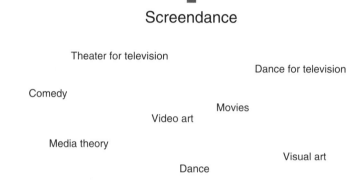

Screen performance

Screendance

Theater for television

Dance for television

Comedy

Movies

Video art

Media theory

Visual art

Dance

Figure 6.3: Genre graph, Douglas Rosenberg
© Douglas Rosenberg

While determining and identifying genre specificity is common practice in the visual arts and film, it is less common in live dance; even so, citations of genre are certainly present. The articulation of live dance by forces both inside and external to the creative circle of practitioners aids us in honing the field into sharp-edged focus in regard to how works of dance circulate and how they are received culturally. It also allows for critics such as Sally Banes and Michael Kirby to refer to "the theory of postmodern dance" as early as 1975.[9] And it allows for artists working with other methodologies to distance themselves from the theory of postmodern dance in order to articulate their own theories and practice. In Banes's *Terpsichore in Sneakers*, she writes:

> When Yvonne Rainer started using the term "postmodern" in the early 1960s to categorize the work she and her peers were doing at the Judson Church and other places, she meant it primarily in a chronological sense. Theirs was the generation that came after modern dance, which was itself originally an inclusive term applied to nearly any theatrical dance that departed from ballet or popular entertainment. By the late 1950s modern dance had refined its styles and its theories, and had emerged as a recognizable dance genre.[10]

Banes parses dance into even smaller and more precise subgenres of practice and recounts the manifestos of each. These lineages and subgenres of dance are primarily embodied via a dancer's training and performance histories, as well as more overt political choices that that dancer may make as to her affiliations with a particular area of practice. By indexing the salient aspect of dance as they pertain to genre and categories, Banes helps to create a discourse about the culture of dance itself.

The methodology by which Banes analyzes dance and its relationship to genre comes from her peripheral vision—what I have called thinking laterally—and appropriates common art world methodologies. Like postmodern dance, video and performance art were part of a movement in the mid 1960s that was catalyzed by concerns about the body as a site of resistance and by new technologies of representation and witnessing. Video and performance art were originally attached to a master narrative stemming from the Fluxus movement, among others, until a critical mass of practitioners began to name their aims and concerns, and to contextualize their creative output in more specific terms.[11] Early video art in many ways mimicked the practice of experimental film, yet in articulating both the material and contextual differences *from film*, video artists and curators were able to begin a discourse specific to the desires of video as an independent art form. Performance art was in its early days was often referred to as "body art," thereby clearly locating the substance or material of the practice within the site of corporeality, inseparable from the body itself. And while body art or performance art might be confused with dance or theater, it was evidently the intent of its practitioners to distance themselves from those narratives and traditions, thus creating a space in which to address their own concerns.

If aggregate areas of art practice are delineated by master categories and further articulated by genres and subgenres, then by the same logic, "dance" is a master category that includes the genres of modern, ballet, tap, contact, and so on. Each of these genres creates its own literature, both by theory and by practice, which defines it as separate from other genres. The literacy of each is thus more or less refined by its practitioners and also by its critics and historians, who collaborate in articulating its provenance and its relationships to other categories and genres of other forms of expression. Though screendance (known also by its various other titles as videodance, dance for camera, etc.) defines itself *in name* and through festivals, screenings, and touring programs, there remains a considerable lack of literacy and scholarship or critical writing about the particular and differing formal and content-based approaches to the practice. In its stead, there is a reliance on shorthand and inferred meaning via the numerous names by which the practice articulates itself.

For instance, while the term "videodance" is used to describe a number of activities involving dance and the moving image, it is, from a linguistic perspective, both quite specific and simultaneously vague. The term implies that the method of recording involves a particular technology (video), which has a documented history as a subset of the visual arts (video art) and as a technology that flows from a particular historical moment (the mid-1960s). Those particularities place whatever may be referred to as videodance in a specific discourse situated in the continuum of the visual arts and a larger discourse around video culture in general. At the same time, the referent "dance" makes the term less precise. That word tells us very little about the provenance of the movement vocabulary, its place within the history of choreographic strategies, or its politics in general. It does not name its place in one of the many specific techniques or schools of movement nor whether it is contemporary or modern, historical, or ballet. Therefore, while videodance is a term that is widely applied, it ultimately does little to illuminate the nature of the work in question. Moreover, other terms are equally misleading or misrepresent the actual materiality of the hybrid of dance and its mediated image in common usage. And like dance itself, *screendance* is a master category with numerous genres and subgenres flowing from it.

Screendance, being a hybrid practice, contains at least two disciplines: dance and screen-based, technologically mediated methods of rendering. In this capacity, it is an overarching master category: screendance implies that the end point of the endeavor is a mediated image of dance on a screen, *any* dance on *any* screen. Indeed, by design and intent, screendance does not imply the materiality of rendering nor does it describe a particular genre of dance practice. It could be shot in film or video, or manifest in a cameraless digital environment. The choreographic language of the work could be modern, postmodern, jazz, ballet, or any other kind of dance. In order to particularize a discussion about a work of screendance, then, it is necessary to further excavate both form and content—the method of rendering as well as the choreographic language. In this way it becomes possible to extrapolate meaning from the common and/or accepted shorthand that is used to describe a range of screendance practice.

We know that the category of visual art has numerous genres and subgenres. Film has genres, dance has genres; therefore hybrids of any two of the above would result in both a genre and have beneath them numerous subgenres. Since screendance is already a hybrid, then, it may be thought of as either a master category or a subgenre of two or more parent genres. As in the case of film and other categories or parent genres, screendance would then propagate its own subgenres as well. These subgenres, given enough of a critical mass may then become a movement. Movements in turn catalyze new genres and are the product of a group of artists who agree on certain general principles and create both artwork and literature that support those principles.

For an example of this phenomenon in the film world, we can look to *Dogma 95*, a manifesto-driven provocation and movement that included the Danish director Lars Von Trier, Thomas Vinterberg, and others who formed the Dogma film collective. The group produced what was called the "Vows of Chastity," a list of ten prescriptions in exacting language that described what a filmmaker could and could not do in order for the film to be considered a *Dogma 95* film.[12] As with most manifestos, it had a short-lived but intense existence. The manifesto inspired a movement that spread beyond film circles into other areas of practice, including the screendance community. Shortly after the "Vows of Chastity" appeared in print, Katrina McPherson, Litza Bixler, and Deveril, all dance filmmakers based in Great Britain, responded to the *Dogma 95* manifesto with their own screendance-specific manifesto, "Dogma Dance":

> YES to the development of dance technique for film—YES to a sharing of knowledge between dance and film—YES to the development of choreographic structure in film—YES to technology which aids rather than hinders—YES to human dancers—YES to the creation of a new genre—YES to safe dancers—YES to the encouragement of dance filmmakers—YES to a new hybrid form.
>
> NO to unsafe dancers—NO to the primacy of equipment and technology over human creativity—NO to the breakdown of choreographic structure—NO to purposeless hierarchies—NO to unbalanced wages—NO to the dominance of film in Dance film.[13]

The stated intent of "Dogma Dance" was to "offer a challenge to dance-film-makers to make their work within the frame-work of 'artistic and production rules,' evolved to encourage the radical development of the medium and the individual's own approach to making work."[14] Illustrating their provocation was a curated screening in London called *Under Your Skin*.[15] The "Dogma Dance" manifesto has echoes of numerous other such statements of purpose in all areas of arts practice, most particularly Yvonne Rainer's *NO manifesto* from 1965 (see chap. 7) but also those by the Futurists and other twentieth-century movements that used such texts to both provoke and catalyze artistic production within a narrowly defined set of parameters.[16]

Manifestos and genres are a way to initiate the organization of data into manageable systems of intellectualized units. The early part of the twentieth century saw countless manifestos from the Dadaists, Surrealists, Futurists, Fluxus artists, and others, which by mid-century had given way to a more coherent naming of styles and genres such as Abstract Expressionism, Pop Art, and later Video Art and Performance Art that had traceable lineages that led back to the manifestos of the earlier part of the century. The manifestos of Dogma Dance, as well as those mentioned above, extend the legacy of artists defining their communities and subsequent experimentation. Screendance, however, has vigorously resisted the kind of scrutiny that comes from naming styles, genres, and approaches to an area of practice.

Ironically, naming such affiliations does not necessarily close down a practice but tends to open it up to new ideas and manifestations. The art historian Henry Sayre refers to the postmodern avant-garde as an art "founded upon contingency, multiplicity and polyvocality." That said, even lacking a coherent and/or recognizable style, art works made in the postmodern era are recognizable and "eminently amenable to a formalist approach [of critique]."[17] Screendance, being a hybrid and performance-based form, would certainly fit under Sayre's description. If we are to include screendance in the discourse of postmodern art practice, however, the task then is to begin to determine how to approach works of screendance in order to read them, name them, critique them, and begin to have a meaningful dialog about them.

The scholar Mark Franko, in "Aesthetic Agencies in Flux: Talley Beatty, Maya Deren and the Modern Dance Tradition in *Study in Choreography for Camera*" offers a reading of Maya Deren's dance film works that gives us a glimpse into the possibilities of viewing such "classic" works through contemporary theoretical lenses.[18] Franko proposes that in Deren's film, both the presence and absence of the dancer Talley Beatty is a "product of the film's manipulation of time and space as well as the vehicle wherein the film itself attains movement. . . . This is what Deren identifies as film dance: 'a dance so related to camera and cutting that it cannot be performed as a unit anywhere but in this particular film.'"[19] Deren's definition of film dance has been the default standard for dance on screen that is *not documentation*, most likely since it was first uttered. That definition cannot be depended on to speak for all works in which movement codified by some metric as "dance" and the technologies of screen media intersect. Franko, in reflecting on Deren's dialectical view of choreography and film, continues:

> For Deren, the limitations of dance arise from the limitations of architecturally defined space germane to live performance. The mobility of the camera and

the manipulations of editing disrupt such limitations and transfigure them. Through the agency of camera and editor, "a whole new set of relationships between dancer and space could be developed."[20]

Deren's statement, although important to the form, overemphasizes the dialectic of dance and media. This dialectical understanding of dance and film is rooted in what Sayre describes as being "eminently amenable to a formalist approach [of critique]." It neutralizes any of the diasporic traces that are brought to bear in either the dance or the media elements, resulting in a visuality that is, in the end, a method of conforming to Modernism's lowest common denominator. Furthermore, it almost completely effaces issues of race, gender, and all of the scattered ephemera that attaches to both sides of the dialectic: the choreographic language and its provenance, the cinematic history and materiality of the methods of inscription. In short, the family tree of such work—its generic heritage—is rendered invisible in favor of a reductive, modernist reading of its formal qualities.

Given the evolution of theoretical discourse in the arts beyond screendance, it is no longer adequate to define a work for the screen by those formal qualities that simply imply that the work could not be created as a live event. Rather, it seems necessary to define new models and critiques related to works of screendance, ones that take into account the commitment of makers to defining the practice in novel and often eccentric ways. In addition, these models should facilitate a deeper understanding of the context by which the work becomes a part of a larger collective discourse on the body's representation on screen, as well as innumerable other concerns that attach to the arts in a contemporary world.

In order to probe the practice and to excavate its genres, my methodology analyzes a work's screenic attributes as well as its vernacular, choreographic attributes: What are the *qualities* of the work that are "of the screen"?[21] What are the *contingencies* that tether the work to the screen, and what are those *histories and theories* that belong to the work in the process? What are the formal qualities of the rendering (which may include style, genre, materiality), and what are the formal qualities of the choreographic language (which may include schools of movement, choreographic vernacular, lineage, and other material associations)? What is the *intent* of the work—that is, what can we infer from the way in which the work is described by title, by the meta-data, and by formal designations such as videodance, dance film, screendance, and the like? And finally, what is the *content* of the work? What are the inferences that can be read by the performance contained within the frame of that which we are consuming, and what are the politics of the work?

In putting these rhetorical suggestions into practice, we look to Viking Eggeling's *Diagonale Symphonie* (1924) as an example of an abstract film that can be probed for its screenic qualities in order to excavate its characteristics and thus assign its relationship to a particular genre.[22] *Diagonale Symphonie* is a silent film in which no humans appear, and yet the film's clear intention is an exploration of the depiction of movement. The film's self-stated purpose is to "discover the basic organization of time intervals in the film medium."[23] It does so by animating objects and shapes across the screen in rhythmic compositional volleys that suggest a kind of musicality, if not a synesthetic representation of music through movement. To more accurately contextualize the film's relative value and to locate the film in a larger interdisciplinary discourse, we need to consider the migration of Eggeling from Germany to Zurich, Switzerland, where he became associated with the Dada movement; the surface qualities of the film (paper cutouts and tinfoil figures photographed a single frame at a time); and also his artistic associations (Hans Richter, Jean Arp, Tristan Tzara, and others). All of this allows us to index those aspects of the film that both separate it from and attach it to other work that flows from a similar set of historical and material circumstances. Thus, we conclude that Eggeling's work is not only informed by the practices of other film artists of the era but also by his associations with the visual artist Arp, and the literary and performative work of Tzara, a central figure of the Dada movement. These affiliations speak to the intent of Eggeling as an artist and create a context for a discourse about his work.

Hans Richter's *Rhythm 23* (1923) is another example of this process. The film—a silent black-and-white study of movement through objects—comes out of the post–World War I cinematic avant-garde that originated in Germany and was composed mainly of painters and photographers.[24] Though visually similar to Eggeling's work, where Eggeling's shapes in motion are linear and graphic, Richter's forms seem more luminous and solid, encroaching on the screen from the edges and moving across the frame or expanding to fill the space until they suggest fleeting moments of monochromatic paintings. Richter's artistic and political affiliations are evident in his own writing at the time and in the visuality of his films.[25] Without elaborating on the diasporic history of Dada and Cubism that is attached to Richter's sense of cinematic materiality and spatial understanding of film, it becomes less possible to accurately place this work within a conversation about screendance. Thus, neither *Diagonale Symphonie* nor *Rhythm 23* are works of screendance per se, (neither filmmaker states such an intent), but an activist curator might include these films within an exhibition of screendance works in order to demonstrate the flexibility of a particular subgenre of screendance practice.[26] It would then fall to the curator to expound a position that supports such an inclusion and how the films might extend our knowledge or understanding of screendance proper.

These examples demonstrate that in order to understand and articulate screen-specific works, it is of value to know the meta-narrative of the work and to "read" both the surface qualities of the film and the meta-knowledge one can attach to the discourse around the work. The films of Eggeling, Richter, and others were materially unlike other art forms. While there is a resemblance to drawing or graphic design, theirs is a set of visual images that is more filmic (or screenic) than graphic, and the sequential appearance of discreet shapes and forms is so deeply embedded in the surface of the film that they are irretrievable as graphic objects in their original form.

Given the attention to surface detail and compositional tools the film-makers employ, the films of Eggeling and Richter might be considered a type of poetic cinema. In a sense, the imagery in both films can be thought of as made solely of insert shots or close-ups. Eschewing the more common practice of cutting such shots into a master shot, the filmmakers deny the sense of narrative/poetic rhythm provided by such editing techniques. As such, neither film could be considered narrative in any traditional sense, but they expose the art of cinema for its own sake rather than as a means of progressing a story by building a lexicon of close-ups, "cut-aways," and symbolic shots of objects in motion separated from a significant master shot. Instead, it is possible to identify what Susan Heyward has described as "poetic symbolism within the narrative" in work that signals its *intent* to tell a story.[27] Ideas about the poetic and the narrative, while often sharing overlapping points of reference may also be seen as two separate and autonomous genres in regard to screendance.

To compare these two simple subgenres useful to the discussion of screendance, then, we might examine the dialog *between* narrative and poetic forms, as these classifications are simultaneously broad and specific. A work in one category may seep into the other, but it is a starting point by which to address both the intent of a work (as Carroll describes) and the result of the work. Erin Brannigan's recent essay offers an insightful dis-course on the use of the close-up in screendance using Miriam King's film, *Dust* as an object of contemplation. Brannigan states that

> one of the projects of dance in the twentieth century has been to reactivate
> or investigate exactly this function of the body: the body as receptive surface
> and responsive organ which can articulate, through the most subtle

micro-movements, the registration of flows of energy, sensory activity and exterior stimuli which occur through and upon the body. When applied to dancefilm, this calls for a reworking of the dominant theories of the cinematic close-up.[28]

While I agree with Brannigan in theory, in "reading" the works she cites as well as others that conform to her theory of *micro-choreographies*, I suggest that the use of the close-up in screendance is most often encountered within a kind of discreet narrativity, one that is *implicit*, made so by an opening combination of shots and edits that lay out a series of juxtapositions by which all subsequent images are referenced.

It is the rare work of screendance that does not begin with a series of shots that are implicitly narrative. In other words, projects often begin and end with the body in motion (or "stillness"), offering no other juxtaposition of place, inanimate objects, locative devices, or musical overlays that contain multiple layers of implied or inferred meaning. In her reading of Miriam King's *Dust*, which she subsequently contrasts with Amy Greenfield's *Element*, Brannigan writes:

> *Dust* begins with a close-up of sand particles blowing across surfaces, creating patterns as they dance and scatter, then hard sand cracks and a hand emerges. This begins a series of close-ups of performer Miriam King's body; her back, fingers crawling across the sand, her eyes which are covered by goggles. King's body emerges through fragments until we see it as a whole, attempting to swim across the sand dunes. The first full close-up of King's face is followed by a close-up of a ticking watch, and then various odd angles render her face strange and unfamiliar. The second half of the film features King's body parts in close-up submerged in black water, the solid form of the figure dissolving in the dark liquid and play of light. . . . This sequence recalls Amy Greenfield's body struggling in thick black mud in *Element* (1973), emerging and disappearing in a study almost entirely shot in close-up. Greenfield's pioneering work in the 1970s combined close-ups of the moving body with intensely motile and loose camera work that "ungrounded" the figure to a radical degree. In both films, the drama is spread across various surfaces, substances and the body of the performer equally, with detailed movements of fingers, limbs and back muscles filling out their intensely visual tales. In such dancefilm examples, the performing body and the close-up have combined to create a new mode of filmic performance.[29]

Brannigan's detailed reading of the two works illuminates the inherent difference between a work that relies on external cinematic devices to ground its meaning and one that does not waver from or capitulate to film's desire for narrative strategies outside of the bodies' own landscape. The opening of Brannigan's description of *Dust* states that it "begins with a close-up of sand particles . . . " Thus, before we even encounter King's body and are allowed to begin our own relationship with its corporeal meaning, we are set up by a series of shots designed to foreground a very particular narrative. She continues, "The first full close-up . . . followed by a close-up of a ticking watch." Again we are brought out of our relationship with the body that Brannigan eloquently describes in her exposition of King's film and into a consideration of the concept of time via a shot of her wristwatch.

Brannigan then notes that "The second half of the film features "King's body parts in close-up submerged in black water . . ., the solid form of the figure dissolving in the dark liquid and play of light" and that "This sequence recalls Amy Greenfield's body struggling in thick black mud. . . ." The difference here is not without consequence. The use of close-up in *Dust* conforms to a historical use of the technique designed to enhance narrativity and thus impose meaning in a manner that is closely aligned with the way in which literary devices are used to tell a story. In *Dust* they are used as a kind of steering device to keep us, the viewers, on track. In Greenfield's *Element*, no such external narrative is present: no literary devices, no juxtapositions of the visual culture of objects or the kind of editing techniques that suggest a narrative outside of the body's experience with itself and its environment. The use of the close-up to contrast the wide shot in *Element* is always limited to the body and the site it inhabits. No other signifiers are present in *Element*; we are free to imagine our own metaphors for the engagement of Greenfield's body to the landscape and her performance within it. In illustrating or engaging in the process of excavating the salient features of a work of screendance, and given the evidence of difference exemplified by the above examples, it becomes possible to parse these works into subgenres, which are themselves contained by the larger category of screendance: King's *Dust* as narrative, and Greenfield's *Element* as poetic, keeping in mind that these delineations are meant as a catalyst for both curating and critical discourse ❺.

At this juncture, there are two points that that might seem to be counterintuitive: the first is that the visual culture of work that transpires at the intersection of dance and screen media is often more dancelike than filmlike: it *looks like dance*. The second is that it *seems* like film. Even the most abstract or "pure" (i.e., non-narrative) choreography tends to capitulate to the desires of cinema, to the desire to be narrative. As Claudia Kappenberg observes, "Almost 30 years after [Amy] Greenfield and 50 years after [Maya]

Deren, much of screendance remains rooted above all in dance traditions"[30] That said, dance resists the *nature* of cinema or video and maintains its identity even if edited and temporally altered. Though embedded in the site of film or video, dance as a realistic technical performance tends to maintain its own nature: again, it still *looks* like dance, or at least the visual culture of dance. Even so, the presentation *of* the visual culture of dance is often embedded in the narrative structures of film in a way that telegraphs a kind of mistrust of the body's ability to transmit its own stories without additional signifiers. Greenfield's *Element* is a possible answer to the rhetorical question that Kappenberg poses: *Does Screendance Need to Look Like Dance?*

To match the sort of hybridity that other interdisciplinary art world practices have achieved, it seems as if screendance must necessarily become more conscious of its own diasporic wanderings, especially as dance becomes more screenic. At the same time, we must begin to create a linguistic apparatus by which to explain the relationships between individual works of screendance and their connections to larger tendencies and movements in the art world in general. This discourse would open new territories of critical thinking in the field as it begins to excavate meaning, histories, materiality, and genre within screendance.

CHAPTER 7

Curating the Practice/The Practice of Curating

Curating and its relationship to screendance might be split into two distinct threads. On the one hand, curation that is focused on the screen and its possibilities for reifying a hybrid and experimental space of activity, and on the other, curating that is focused on the representation and inscription of dance in order to reinforce distinct and entrenched notions of choreography in their migration to screen space. In the first example dance is but one element in the construction of a performative screenic space, purposefully subsumed into such space in order to engage its specificities. In the second example of curation, its gestures are predetermined to retain the authority of dance as a discrete artform within screenic space. Each approach performs a specific agenda and reinforces a particular ideology. The practice of curating screendance, given these two different paths, might result in either a kind of triumph of dance over the desires of media or the disappearance of dance into the space *of* media. In the former, dance maintains its authority over the method of inscription and circulation and in the latter the gesture of curating would, quite possibly in the end, result in reinforcing screendance as an autonomous art form. Here, the sort of curating that might take as its mission, an opening outward of the gestalt of screendance, would ultimately dilute the "purity" of dance, (if such a thing exists) in favor of a layering of elements that each sacrifice their own autonomy in service to a new hybrid form. Screendance by its very nature must consistently and constantly address its own bifurcation and the tension between two distinctly oppositional forces; the desire of dance to forestall its own appropriation, and the desire of the screen to consume any and all gestures into its own materiality.

The desire for dance to maintain its autonomy in relation to media, whether intentional or not, is underscored by the titles of many of the texts that address the relationship of dance to the screen: *Dancefilm, Choreography and the Moving Image* (Erin Brannigan), *Dance on Screen* (Sherril Dodds), and *Envisioning Dance on Film and Video* (Judy Mitoma) telegraph their concerns for the autonomy of dance as an art form in the structure of their titles. The authors of *Parallel Lines: Media Representations of Dance* (Stephanie Jordan and Dave Allen) go a step farther in their introduction as they note that their book will address the questions of, "What is dance?" and "How should dance be represented" on screen. Furthermore, they state specifically that the book is "aimed principally at a dance audience." Such a conversation enforces a closed circuit discourse and negates disparate voices from other disciplines that might illuminate the relationship between dance and media.

By contrast, Andre Lepecki in *Exhausting Dance: Performance and the Politics of Movement*, telegraphs his intent to untether or unmoor dance from its entrenched identities by attempting to "address the choreographic outside the proper limits of dance."[1] Clearly, Lepecki is writing from a distinctly different point of view than the authors of the texts mentioned earlier. However, Lepecki's gesture of asking dance studies to "step into other artistic fields and to create new possibilities for thinking relationships between bodies, subjectivities, politics, and movement" is, at its core, an act of curating.[2] In the form of a text, Lepecki gathers together examples of performative conceptual threads in the framework of artists disparate from those relied on by dance history and creates a kind of virtual exhibition that is both textual and performative. Such a method may be seen as a model for screendance as well.

The practice of curating in general comes from an art model in which an individual or team attempts to create meaning from a group of artworks. According to Geoff Cox and Joasia Krysa, curation, "subjective and taxonomic by nature, can be viewed as the practice of constructing meaning by exerting control through selection, clever arrangement, labeling, interpretation and so on."[3] Thus, meaning accrues via the relationship of one object or image or film to another as seen through numerous cultural lenses and frames of reference. In this capacity, curating dance film and video is a way of constructing narratives about the field of screendance that may be otherwise invisible or absent.

Curating may also serve to interrogate individual works of screendance, collective, individual or group practice, and to actively shape and comment upon the field in general. It creates a foundation for criticality as it frames and groups individual works around issues of content, form, or myriad other concerns. Curating and criticality are thus linked and synergistically contribute to an elevated discussion about meaning, purpose, form, and content in the field of screendance. Yet it seems that curating, in its truest sense is largely absent from the screendance festival circuit and from screendance exhibition in general.[4] The lack of curatorial activism leads to a malaise, even disengagement on the part of both makers and spectators that diminishes the potential of screendance as an artform.

As the field of screendance increases in popularity and more festivals emerge around the world, it is important to consider questions relating to both curatorial prerogative and to the ways festivals are programmed. Festivals are the conduits through which most people view screendance, though it is often unclear how a festival builds its public programs. Is there a jury, an individual curator, perhaps a combination of both? What is the difference between a curated or juried screening and one that is "programmed," and what are the concerns and missions of each?

The gap between curation and programming leads one to consider a series of rhetorical questions that shape this chapter:

- What responsibilities do programmers and directors of screendance festivals have in regard to defining the field?
- Can curating function as a kind of critical thinking?
- What part might curators play in creating intelligent and thoughtful programming that articulates a distinct point of view that sets one festival apart from another?
- What does it mean to curate a program of dances for the screen?
- What historical precedents are there to be found in fine art or experimental cinema models?
- How might curating function as historical documentation?
- Does an articulately curated program function as a text for understanding the form?
- How might curating shape a dialogue about entertainment and the relationship of media to dance?
- What might curated program allow for that program chosen by other means might not?
- Can curating define a model for criticality?
- How might curating help to enunciate genres in the field?

These questions, while somewhat rare in discussions surrounding screendance, are significantly more prevalent in the visual arts.[5] Liz Wells, a UK-based curator, makes the following statement:

> Exhibition involves imposition of order on objects, brought into a particular space and a specific set of relations with one another. The ordering may be in

accord with established classifications and habits of display or may challenge conventions; but is necessarily rhetorical in calling attention to artefacts brought together to be subjected to visual scrutiny. Exhibition commands visual attentiveness. This is taken for granted in museum and gallery studies.[6]

Curating is not simply about choosing. It is a proactive practice, which by its very nature contains in equal parts academic/pedantic/scholarly and teaching components. One undertakes a high degree of responsibility as a curator, not only to the work but also to the culture of the art form in general, its historical provenance, its way forward, and its flow of inter-related tributaries: interdisciplinarity and intertextuality. Curating is a platform for strong statements and is quite different than arranging or programming. It relies on a set of strategies that are intended to speak back to the form very directly, and in many cases it attempts to move the form in a particular direction. Curating is also about using works of art to make the definitive statement that something exists outside the form, such as disability, gender, and the like.

Programming, which is the more prevalent model in screendance festivals, is a kind of showcase, not unlike a dance concert that has multiple choreographers on the same bill. The underlying similarities between artists sharing the same program may be vague or not entirely apparent; often they appear together for reasons wholly outside of the content or style of their work, reasons that may be pragmatic or otherwise. Programming is the inverse of curating; it is a cross between the way film festivals and some dance events are often conceived. In both cases it follows an entertainment model and therefore has an agenda that is colored by audience expectations. Programming may be done around a theme, but it is still a different undertaking than curation, with a markedly different outcome.

The curator, though not exempt from the business of art, generally operates within a different set of expectations. The curator assumes responsibility for the gestalt of the exhibition that itself further iterates a particular point of view by using works of art as texts, which by implication or inference create collective meanings.[7] Curating implies that a third party has an active role in choosing and arranging the work in a program in such a way as to create a meta-narrative between pieces, between artists, and between the content present in the work the audience ultimately sees. According to the curator Paul O'Neill's essay, "The Curatorial Turn: From Practice to Discourse": "Group exhibitions are ideological texts which make private intentions public. In particular, it is the temporary art exhibition that has become the principal medium in the distribution and reception of art; thus, being the principle agent in debate and criticism about any aspect of the visual arts."[8] While O'Neill refers specifically to the visual arts, festival screenings are essentially group exhibitions; as such, the thrust of his statement is on point. The role of the curator is more than active; it is *proactive* in that the curator's job is to seek out work that supports a thesis, a thesis that the curator seeks to introduce into the culture of the art form (screendance for instance) in order to create a conversation about the art form itself. In other words, the curated exhibition endeavors to create a gestalt based on the relationships between individual pieces, amplifying meaning beyond the scope of a single artwork. In this way, the spectator's engagement is deepened as well. Curated exhibitions or screenings catalyze new ideas about genre, style, trends, and historical provenance, and these also serve as a text for a larger discourse about the art form or about issues that are of concern to the curator (political, cultural, or other). With screendance, curation elevates the practice to one in which rigorous interrogation of dance and its relationship to the screen, of dance itself, of issues of representation and agency and beyond, vibrate across the entire practice and the community of practitioners. If we add critical writing and reportage to this mix, the field begins to look like a serious creative social space in which important and meaningful dialogs may take place, which will ultimately benefit the field. It also begins to address issues of artistic citizenship, that is, the involvement of both makers and consumers of such creative work in defining the field, reinforcing a kind of synergistic community practice.

Both dance and media have become culturally ubiquitous. Reality television has turned its attention toward dance in various forms: dance appears on the Academy Awards shows and in commercials; one can see dance in numerous incarnations on YouTube and other media sites; and there are any number of movies that foreground dance to tell a story, often one about triumph over class or social status. These representations of dance on film and video have certainly affected the way that dance is represented in the genre of practice that we call screendance. The trend toward spectacle, lavish production, and virtuosic performance is clearly visible in the work one encounters on the international screendance festival circuit. The oscillation between what is often historically referred to as high and low culture, or as the postwar critic Clement Greenberg framed it, "avant-garde and kitsch," is a constant in art history. But in the current mediatized culture, where the gap between life and art has become porous and boundaries that once existed to delineate one practice from another have been largely dissolved, the blending of these disparate elements exerts an undeniable pressure on the arts to keep up and to compete with a visual culture that is, at times, overwhelmingly frantic.

Greenberg used the term "kitsch" to identify a kind of esthetically impoverished art-product that, in pretending to be high art, attracted those who wished to align themselves with high culture in order to signal class status. He points out the importance of relational proximity in a way that also illuminates curatorial practice:

> It appears to me that it is necessary to examine more closely and with more originality than hitherto the relationship between aesthetic experience as met by the specific—not the generalized—individual, and the social and historical contexts in which that experience takes place. What is brought to light will answer, in addition to the question posed above, other and perhaps more important questions.[9]

Greenberg asks the reader to focus more closely on the context from which the work of art emanates, in order to make judgments on the esthetic value as well as the cultural value of that work of art. Context is also the impetus for much curatorial practice and a factor in creating intertextual relationships between works of art: groupings of works that emanate from similar creative impulses often addressing similar issues of form or content.

Greenberg, as well as other theorists of the modern era including Theodor Adorno, framed the avant-garde and kitsch as opposites.[10] Adorno's argument against kitsch was that it was merely a product of the "culture industry" and subject to the needs of a marketplace, which desired entertainment above all else. Adorno held that true art should be both subjective and challenging; Greenberg proposed that art should aspire to a higher calling. In his essay Greenberg notes that "the avant-garde itself, already sensing the danger [of "superficial phenomena"], is becoming more and more timid every day that passes."[11] He felt that it was the duty of the avant-garde to battle against the diminishment of art that the cultural acceptance of kitsch enabled. Indeed, the avant-garde, for him, was a point of resistance.

As postmodernism evolved in the 1980s, the once clear-cut boundaries between the avant-garde and kitsch became blurred as *irony* entered the vernacular. The embrace of irony (as well as techniques of appropriation) led to a praxis that embraced popular culture and often invited mass consumption and mass media practices, thus elevating kitsch to the discourse of high art. In the world of dance and media, the allure of television and its wider audiences has greatly enticed makers of screendance. The legacy of that enticement is a kind of work that mimics the spectacle of both television and Hollywood in its scale, production values, and often its content.

In the UK, commissions for dance films through the BBC and other agencies has produced extremely televisual work. In Canada, Bravo!FACT has set a benchmark for production quality in short dance films, linked to the production values of television and cinema. More recently, though they are not alone in this observation, works such as *The Rain,* by Pontus Lidberg (Sweden, 2007), and *The Cost of Living* (UK, Lloyd Newson, 2004), both screened to much acclaim in numerous festivals, feature the kind of high-end production values that resemble mainstream commercial film and advertising more than experimental or avant-garde endeavors. Media's surface qualities telegraph its affiliations and provenance often as much as does the content of a work for the screen.

While the content of such work may be provocative, the work circulates culturally through mainstream broadcast television outlets and dance film festivals rather than in the underground and/or marginalized spaces often associated with avant-garde film and performance. Broadcast television, antithetical to experimental filmmakers and early video artists' ideas about the spaces in which media art should inhabit, has now become the aspiration of many directors and choreographers. This phenomenon follows the funding sources in the UK and Canada, as well as other countries, where one finds commissioning funds flowing from entities attached to television stations such as the BBC, which have featured so-called arts programming. As such, screendance, in a broadcast venue, has been largely ignored by scholars and critics of media, whose focus is more often on work found in the cinema or in museums and galleries. Television's proclivity for creating juxtapositions of media and programming, which are only marginally related, has carried into the festival circuit as well, to the extent that often "dance" is the only factor linking one screened work to another. Television has also imposed its qualities and sense of space to the internet as well. While discreet viewing of dance media is possible on the web, those products tend to conform to television's pre-existing parameters of production and distribution. While such streaming media may be available "on demand" it is mostly the product of a production that is not specifically created for the web, but rather intended as a multi-purpose product for festival screening, television or any other output.

Although modern dance has addressed its own existential crises throughout the twentieth century and beyond, splintering the practice into sub-genres grouped around particular manifestos and identities, screendance has yet to follow suit. Screendance in its most contemporary manifestation is a part of the postmodern condition, using the tools of fragmentation particular to postmodern representation. As such, it seems logical to expect that screendance should also adopt the theoretical underpinnings of postmodern thinking, resulting in a body of work that would both venture into the territory of postmodern content and simultaneously critique the practice as well. Under this assumption, screendance would ultimately break with modernist ideas and manifestations of spectacle.

There are multiple trends in screendance production and, as is often the case, one can identify a pendulum swing away from one dominant paradigm and toward another. For example, in the 1990's the ubiquity of screendance based on spectacle and virtuosity spurred work that might be described as intimate, socially conscious, humble, and thought provoking. This is work that at its core comes from a conceptual impulse, which is antithetical to spectacle. It often trades the veneer of polished surfaces for the more difficult gestalt of content *and* form. Work such as *Outside In* (1994), directed by Margaret Williams and choreographed by Victoria Marks; *Boy* (1995) by Peter Anderson and Rosemary Lee; and *Elegy* (1993), directed by Chris Graves and choreographed and performed by Douglas Wright are screendance projects that probe the way in which we value bodies and performance through an intimate humanistic approach to media practice. Furthermore, they raise substantive questions about the form and practice of screendance. The bodies we encounter in *Outside In, Boy,* and *Elegy*—some of which are disabled, diseased, or lacking voice—are bodies from the margins of culture, often without agency or representation. And while we may encounter similar bodies in work that tends toward spectacle, the politics of each film along with issues of form and surface quality must finally play a part in the analysis of the work.

In screendance festivals around the world, the dominant model is a programmed festival.[12] Here, the films are often selected from a call for entries and put into a screening order over the course of one or more days and nights. The programmed festival model is one that generally eschews a body of work by a single artist created over time, in favor of the most recent "cutting-edge" and/or timely works, and one that might be described as *populist*. While the festival model currently dominates the exhibition of screendance, however, this has not always been the case, at least in the United States. Seminal exhibitions of screendance work have taken place outside of the festival model since the earliest days of video. One of the earliest media collectives, Video Free America in San Francisco, produced and curated work from the late 1960s through the 1980s. The Pacific Film Archive in Berkeley, California, screened curated programs, as did independent curators in makeshift venues, underground cinemas, and later in dance spaces such as the Dance Theater Workshop in New York. These examples grew out of many fertile and collaborative efforts between the visual arts, performance, and film/video practices.

Such collaborative efforts produce work that creates liminal spaces between genres, which serve as containers for collaborative and interdisciplinary practice. Yvonne Rainer's work often inhabits this space between genres.[13]Her well-known manifesto is often read in the context of postmodern dance; in it she articulates a position regarding a theory that has been overlooked for its significance to the field of screendance. In *NO Manifesto* (1965), the choreographer/filmmaker states:

> No to spectacle no to virtuosity no to transformations and magic and make believe no to glamour and transcendency of the star image no to the heroic no to the anti-heroic no to trash imagery no to involvement of performer or spectator no to style no to camp no to seduction of spectator by the wiles of the performer no to eccentricity no to moving or being moved. [14]

This quotation may be read as a prescription for early dance film, including work by the American Amy Greenfield. In a quintet of films made between 1970 and 1973, Greenfield reifies Yvonne Rainer's manifesto in films such as *Encounter* (1970), *For God While Sleeping* (1970), *Transport* (1971), *Dirt* (1971), and *Element* (1973). For Greenfield, technical dancing is irrelevant; rather, the mise-en-scène of bodies in real, physical, traumatic, and repetitive motion lies at the core of her cinematic exploration. In *Transport,* for example, we see a group of people, not performers or dancers but individuals, who can only be immediately identified as humans engaged in a visceral set of tasks undertaken with deep conviction. We see the group carrying a member aloft over rugged terrain, until exhaustion sets in and then another member is lifted above their heads and the process repeats, and yet throughout there is no artifice and little evidence of the camera's alteration of reality. As in Rainer's manifesto, there is no cinematic magic in these early films, no glamour, and certainly no transformation. They are a product of their material and formal qualities, and nothing more is implied or inferred. Neither the movers nor the film are virtuosic. The film is a moment in time, an intervention of camera and recording device into a mindful version of what Allan Kaprow might call "childsplay."[15] *Transport* thus breaks down expectations of both performance and the art of filmmaking. In Greenfield's early work, nothing and everything happens simultaneously. Her work is a connective thread from dance to what would later become known as performance art; it also connects to conceptual and minimal art. In a time of great change in the broader art world, Greenfield's films are a flashpoint for hybridity within the context of an evolving esthetic of screendance. They are not dance, but neither can one argue successfully that they are not *not*-dance. They are exhortations to reconsider the nature of dance, community, and cinema.

The work of the American filmmaker and intermedia artist Elaine Summers echoes both Rainer and Kaprow, with forays into live dance performance. Summers was a member of the Judson Dance Theater in New York, the seminal group considered central to the foundation of postmodern dance in the early 1960s.[16] The group, which grew out of a dance composition class with Robert Dunn, included such luminaries as Trisha Brown, Steve Paxton, and David Gordon. The Judson group questioned the very nature of dance and its practice, opening the door to a new set of possibilities, including dance on film and video, and dance in a mediated environment.[17] Summers worked extensively with projected film and images in a dance environment, beginning as early as the first Judson concert in 1962; in addition, she made freestanding dance films. She founded the Experimental Intermedia Foundation in New York as well as her own dance/intermedia company, the Elaine Summers Dance and Film Company, which toured experimental multimedia works from the 1970s on. Summers's work in multimedia, from its earliest stages, made dance an element in a kind of *gesamtkunstwerk* of imagery; this in turn became a model for generations of other artists whose work involved synthesizing dancing bodies into an electronic field of activity. Her films, including *In the Absence and the Presence* (1985), *Iowa Blizzard* (1973), and *Two Girls Downtown Iowa* (1973), deconstruct dance and *re*-present it as formalist, abstract imagery that suggests, but does not demonstrate, dance. Summers's use of movement in those seminal films was often excruciatingly slow; it asked the viewer to forego expectations of more traditional elements of "choreography" in favor of a gestalt of cinematic motion. The resonance of her approach is evident in many subsequent dance films, and even more so in the very idea of intermedia or multimedia dance activity.

In 1983, out of their respective engagements with the art, film, and dance milieus, Amy Greenfield and Elaine Summers curated and produced the important Filmdance Festival that took place at the Public Theater in New York, with more than one hundred films and filmed sequences scheduled in twenty-one different programs. They also produced a slim black catalog, highly prized among students and scholars of the genre, containing essays by filmmakers and choreographers. Both Summers and Greenfield—as well as James Byrne, who curated screenings at Dance Theater Workshop (DTW)—were artists first, though artists that were interdisciplinary and often worked outside of the discipline of dance. Byrne's press release for "Eyes Wide Open" in 1989 at DTW states:

Featured in the program are dance films and videos that demonstrate bracingly innovative approached to constructing cinematic choreography from disparate and minimal movement sources. All of these works strive to create new forms and structures for the presentation of a screen reality dealing with the human figure and movement. None of the films deal with a traditional approach to filming dance. . . . This fascinating selection of new works presents a range of possibilities that push and expand the edges of dance video.[18]

Byrne's curator's statement puts his agenda out in front of the work and creates a context for viewing. It makes evident that the selection of work both troubles and questions the nature of the form. It also operates as a challenge to both makers and curators to answer by way of further exhibitions.

In the catalog *Filmdance 1890s–1983*, Amy Greenfield writes:

This catalog sets out to discuss the nature of filmdance. Each writer in the catalog was free to choose his or her own subject. No writer knew the specific viewpoints of the others. Therefore, the articles present varying, sometimes opposing, definitions, theories, and discussions on the nature of Filmdance. . . . The artists who responded to the invitation to write have made statements either on their own films or on their theories of filmdance. In setting down their thoughts, they further help to articulate the varying and changing nature of filmdance.[19]

James Byrne and Amy Greenfield each make their case for curatorial prerogative, but in their statements both also point to the larger needs and desires of the field. Their statements articulate a methodology for how the work might circulate conceptually. Likewise, the festival model also creates a context for viewing and sets parameters for discourse; however, it often lacks a thesis and may be driven by desires and needs that are unclear in regard to a desired outcome.

Institutionalizing such a lack of clarity results in an increasingly difficult climate for critique and social change via the practice. Historically, all art movements have in some way critiqued their own institutions through exhibitions, publications, or other means. In order for art to exert its ability to instigate cultural change, it cannot allow itself to become fallow or content with the status quo. As screendance festivals (and to some extent, broadcast outlets and streaming media sites) are the dominant mode of exhibition for the form, much contemporary work is modeled, consciously or not, on the demands and criteria of those exhibition and screening opportunities. Screendance festivals, in many cases, function more as agents for the distribution of dance on film than as arbiters of any sort of intellectual or critical "moment" in the evolution of the form. Although this model may be an entertaining adjunct to theater dance, it is void of the criticality that would help to give the practice a voice outside of its own community. It is precisely due to this issue that the field needs the kind of polyvocality in which artists from non-Western or other self-defined (feminist, queer, hybrid, other) cultures speak through their work both in theory and in practice and also the reason why curatorial activism is so important at this moment. What artists like Deren, Greenfield, Summers, and others achieved was a complete rupture with the culture of their time, a break with Hollywood musicals and with documentation of virtuosic dancing as film art. Their work should not be construed, therefore, only as a nostalgic looking-backwards to the "roots" of screendance but as a model of engagement and activism.

The term "screendance" is roughly the equivalent to the term "painting." In other words, it describes a practice by its formal characteristics in the broadest terms. The articulation of a practice beyond those terms requires a subset of language that begins to speak about the work in more particular terminology. That is, terminology that begins to allude to style, content, affiliations, histories, provenance, and lineage, as well as movements— whether art historical, dance historical, or something else. To have a show of "painting" without articulating the frame of the specific works in the exhibition (new abstraction, color field, pop, etc.) or at least their resonant affiliations would be extremely rare in the art world at large. In such a scenario, it is the job of the curator to choose the paintings for inclusion and to subsequently create a statement in the form of a catalog essay or some other text that lays out a rationale and a frame or lens for the show. Further, that essay would address *why* the group of paintings is gathered and arranged in a particular way, as well as identify the connective tissue between the works and their intertexts (what do these works have to say to each other and to the form?) and perhaps speak about the form itself. What is the state of affairs in painting" Does this work indicate a change in course for the practice? Does it restate an existing course? While curation per se is rare in the dance world, it has existed from time to time as artist-led practice (the Judson Church group being one of the most memorable), in the gravitational pull of downtown dance in New York, and in the self-organizing nature of postmodern dance as it established itself as an alternative to modern dance.

In the screendance festival model, we often see a small group of films repeatedly screened from festival to festival. The similarity in style and approach at international festival selections is often striking. To revisit the painting analogy, these trends might be recognized as movements or styles and named (Abstract Expressionist, Realism, and so forth) in order to explicate their generic sources. To use a musical analogy, there might be a particular approach to making screendance that could be referred to as "classical," in which we might group works by artists through the mid-twentieth century. Alternately, taking a cue from the visual arts, other sub-genres might include the designations, "formalist," "narrative" or "popular" to delineate commonalities and concerns within various approaches to constructing works for the screen. Works could be further delineated by materiality, surface qualities, subject, choreographic language, and political content. As makers and curators, we have the ability to illuminate new ideas about our field through discourse commensurate to other established modes of art practice. By curating an alternative to the strand of work that seems too ubiquitous, and by creating an essay or rationale that frames it, we can illuminate another set of possibilities and move the field forward.

Discussions of screendance often cite Hollywood musicals and other film/dance hybrids as part of the discourse.[20] But screendance is more than a subset of Hollywood musicals, music video, or other such amalgams of the entertainment industry. Screendance has not clearly established itself as a field of practice distinct and separate from other these and other genres, and this is precisely the problem that can be addressed by curation and certainly by critical writing. By vocalizing difference and articulating specificity in the practice, it may be possible to move the field toward other models found in the visual arts and elsewhere. The present scenario in the screendance environment, in which festival models prevail and in which films are often referred to as "the best" of a given year or "the best" festival choices and subsequently populate other festivals, creates a model that is self-perpetuating. If these *are* the best films, then might it be logical as a viewer and maker to emulate the style of work that is being granted such status? Again, the desire for success or validation, competition if you will, drives the practice thus reinforcing the status quo. If, instead, festival programs and exhibitions of work in other venues were curated to make a number of statements that exceed the films themselves and engage broader dialogs about the culture at large, about media, about humanism—then perhaps screendance practice might be able to move toward the gravitas of the art world proper.

Dialogs surrounding screendance often describe and articulate elements of the practice that are less about stating what it is *not* than stating what it *is*. Screendance is often described as "not like Hollywood musicals" or "different than music videos," or "not simply dance documentation," but a point of differentiation does not constitute a genre. A close example would be "performance art," a term widely used beginning in the 1970s for a practice that shifted the site of objectification from materials found in the world to the material of the body itself. Performance art differentiated the site of art practice from the material site of painting or sculpture: it named the practice "art" and the genus "performance." The term has, since then, fallen out of favor and been replaced by the much less cumbersome "performance" to describe both practice and genus. This is similar to the evolution of the term "rock 'n' roll," which differentiated the new sound from the old. First, the term was shorthanded to "rock music," and now of course we simply need to say "rock" to be understood. This evolution of language relies on a preexisting set of conditions and a certain amount of connoisseurship. But the cultural understanding of performance art, as well as conceptual art, minimalism (and the list goes on), was articulated in practice by curators (sometimes by artist/curators). It was often simultaneously described and critiqued by writers and artists themselves. It was curation, though, that provided the visualization and the critical mass of objects arranged within a particular logic for both viewer and critic to ruminate, meditate, and reflect upon. Similarly, in regard to screendance, it is curation that will begin to excavate genres, patterns, and modalities within the practice.

So why is curating important to screendance? Curating creates a sense of identity. Curating dance film and video is a way of constructing narratives about the field of screendance that may be otherwise invisible or absent. It is also a way to interrogate individual works of screendance, collective, individual, or group practice and to actively shape and comment upon the field in general. However, a further question to consider is this: "What does the curator want from you, the audience?" What the audience might offer in turn is a kind of feedback loop in which the efforts of the curator or programmer are reflected, considered, and responded to in a thoughtful and focused manner. The audience embodies the work and moves it out into the larger culture of dance and media, into their own practice and into their social situations through discourse and reiteration. In this model, there is a partnership implied, a relationship between makers, curators, festivals, and audiences that might move the field forward in a way that elevates both the work and the critical discourse surrounding it. In talk given in 2009 at the first International Screendance Network meeting in Brighton[21] the film historian Ian Christie invoked the well-known quotation by film critic André Bazin: "cinema has not yet been invented!"[22] Claudia Kappenberg has suggested a revision of Bazin's original thusly: "Screendance Has Not Yet Been Invented".[23] Such a revision suggests that Bazin's call to action on behalf of cinema is equally worth considering on behalf of screendance. If one project of curation is to bring clarity to a collective undertaking such as screendance, then perhaps the project of curation is, in the end, to finally *invent* screendance.

CHAPTER 8

"Seeing is Forgetting the Name of the Thing One Sees," or Connoisseurship in Screendance

The title of this chapter refers to Lawrence Weschler's 1982 book, *Seeing is Forgetting the Name of the Thing One Sees*, which explores the work of the West Coast conceptual artist Robert Irwin.[1] The phrase is invoked here to imply the phenomena of dislocation that occurs in the face of Irwin's early work with light and space. His conceptual installations of the 1970's used pure light to alter the viewer's perception of the space it inhabited to the extent that one often misplaced the language necessary to accurately describe such an experience. On the one hand, the viewer knew their experience through corporeal engagement or embodiment of the work but on the other hand, one often lacked the proper cognition to turn such corporeal knowledge into language. One project of connoisseurship as it pertains to screendance specifically, is to unravel the Gordian knot of perception and articulation, encourage remembering and further to enunciate what one experiences.

The word *connoisseurship* comes from the Latin *cognoscere*, "to know," which on the surface seems to be at least one function of an audience: to *know* what has been collected and put before them. Knowing implies understanding, or at the least, experiencing an event or phenomena with some sense of intimacy. There are of course, at least two types of "knowing": the embodied, experiential way of knowing, and the intellectual, critical knowing generally associated with scholarship. These two approaches are the polar ends of a spectrum across which we come to understand and differentiate works of art. Susan Sontag, speaking about image making in *On Photography*, states: "Picture-taking has been interpreted in two entirely different ways: either as a lucid and precise act of knowing, of conscious intelligence, or as a pre-intellectual, intuitive mode of encounter."[2] In short, one manifests itself as an intellectual response; the other as a sort of "gut reaction."

Both intellectual responses and gut reactions may be relied upon in order to defend matters of relative taste and style, but discerning the relative or quantifiable value of works of screendance with any sort of authority *beyond* personal preference (gut reaction) requires certain particular knowledges. These include the histories of similar work, the framing devices and context of the exhibition or broadcast venue, and the author's intent. When these elements are obfuscated or obscured, the object itself— the screendance—becomes unknowable beyond its formal or material qualities, and thus beyond the limitations of "pre-intellectual" knowledge. This manifests as a kind of resistance, as the objects presented for contemplation collectively resist knowing (or connoisseurship). In a field that is unsure of its own histories and boundaries, or whose parameters have not been adequately excavated, that *unknowing* is further exacerbated and connoisseurship, as a path toward greater knowledge and discourse, is impaired.[3]

One of the stated intents for this book is to create a foundation of criticality for the field in order to attribute genre, stylistic affiliation, or other recognizable markers to works of screendance; in short, a discourse that is separate from market forces and is foremost concerned with clarifying the field and its specificities. From such a foundation we may begin to scaffold a number of practices that will illuminate difference. One of the elements contained within such a scaffold might be thought of as auteurism, that which marks one filmmaker's project as unique and separate from another. In *Engaging the Moving Image*, Noël Carroll writes:

> A leading aim of auteurism is to differentiate one body of films from others—to say what is unique about the work of a given filmmaker. In this way, auteurism is connected to connoisseurship. This is not to say that auteurism need lack a certain explanatory dimension; the auteurist may explain how certain vistas of John Ford's westerns—are expressive of his point of view about American History. The auteurist's project, however, in terms of its "bottom line," remains tied to differentiating one filmmaker's oeuvre from those of others.[4]

This differentiation is the basis for knowing not just the provenance of the film itself but also the context within which a particular film may be situated, either by the maker or the consumer. Context provides a *way in* to critical discourse and such discourse is a means by which a nascent field may begin to understand and situate itself in a larger context.

Auteurism in the context of screendance has gone largely unexamined, though the histories of dance in general are written around and through auteurs such as Martha Graham, Merce Cunningham, Paul Taylor, and others all the way back to Isadora Duncan. Auteurism in dance has led to recognizable choreographic voices as well as equally recognizable styles, genres, and movements in the field. Yet, screendance resists such excavations and descriptions of similar artistic and conceptual tendencies. Perhaps this is a product of the way in which screendance is circulated and managed. It is, nonetheless, antithetical to the nature of much of the work we encounter in festivals and elsewhere, one strand of which may be cinematic or televisual and another which often tends to be small of scale, handmade by an individual or small team of makers. Work of the second type, is reminiscent of the earliest days of cinema and particularly the work-flow of George Méliès, who as Elizabeth Ezra describes, "was an *auteur* in the true sense—in that he was personally involved in every aspect of production."[5] It was a gesture that made Méliès's films recognizable and particular, and what allows the viewer to mark a film as his. It is found subsequently in what Chirstinn Whyte positively identifies as a strand of "amateurism" emerging from mid-twentieth-century, North American, avant-garde film artists including Maya Deren, Stan Brakhage, and Jonas Mekas.[6] Yet, while Méliès, Deren, and others are heralded for their individual contributions to the cinematic arts, auteurism (and the subsequent migration toward connoisseurship) has yet to be adequately identified and or embraced in the milieu of screendance.

The festival screening model dominates the way in which screendance circulates and is received or consumed by audiences; as such, it is the single most generative site of community in the field. However, festivals are not transparent, neutral disseminations of content. The focal point for the audience as the lights go down—the screen itself—is a space fraught with competing desires, upon which is projected not only the ephemeral images of mediated bodies but often the equally fraught desires of the audience. Festivals too are formed out of the desires of funding agencies, managers, directors, entrepreneurs, artists, and others engaged with the process of creating a venue for audiences to view screendance.

Complicating these dynamics, the behavior of audiences is not random: rather, it is learned. How audiences view and receive screendance—in short, spectatorship is in part a phenomena of the behavior of the host institution. In other words, the audience performs its role based to a certain extent on the set of circumstances set forth by the institution and by other cultural institutions familiar to the audience. Audience and spectator are decidedly different performances, with considerable theory dedicated to each. On this, Patrick Phillips writes, "Audiences are seen as constructed by mass-media institutions and exist in a dependent relationship to these institutions."[7] In other words, the audience is the mass of people who are by one means or another drawn to the event, who fill the seats, and who form a kind of performative community for the duration of the event. Again, "The audience disappears when the lights go out. Spectatorship theories . . . kick in at this point, with the audience de-aggregated into individuals alone before the screen."[8]

Screendance is situated in the applause arts, but often what the audience is applauding is unclear. Is it the dancing, the filmmaking, or some combination thereof? Audiences generally do not respond to film screenings by applauding as they do with the live arts. Yet, screendance audiences, perhaps channeling the protocols of live dance, *do* applaud. As screendance in its institutionalized form is most often contextualized by its relationship to dance, the protocols and traditions of concert dance have migrated to screendance and embedded themselves into its viewing and reception practices.

Such traditions of viewing further contextualize the reception of screendance. If such institutions as screendance festivals promote the genre as an extension of dance practice—for example, "dance on film"—then the audience is likely to self-select: patrons who seek a historically understood definition of dance will attend, expecting the dance they desire on the screen at which they are looking. If institutions assume the desires of their audience and endeavor to meet these desires preemptively, then connoisseurship builds around a set of "texts" predetermined by the institution. To a large extent, the examples of screendance put forth by presenting institutions determine a "canon," which becomes inscribed through repetition. It is, however, a canon by default, a passive canon, and as such circulates and embeds itself onto the field, eventually becoming impermeable and resistant to critical analysis. As terms like "classic" or "groundbreaking" begin to attach to certain works without the benefit of critical scholarship or theoretical analysis, modernist tropes of taste and populism are perpetuated. It is commonly assumed in the postmodern era that such canons and tropes are no longer stable or viable, and contemporary connoisseurship would acknowledge that hybrid practices such as screendance are sites that invite volatility. Further, through curatorial prerogative, genres and movements may be illuminated and/or illustrated. Certainly, festivals and presenters might counterprogram in order to illuminate other examples and practices within the field; but because festivals do not generally differentiate between genres of dance or genres of screendance, the possibility of an active, informed connoisseurship in audiences is greatly diminished.

Connoisseurship in general has fallen from favor in the twenty-first century, but there is much to be gleaned from an informed connoisseurship. Mark K. Smith notes that connoisseurship:

> involves the ability to see, not merely to look. To do this we have to develop the ability to name and appreciate the different dimensions of situations and experiences, and the way they relate one to another. We have to be able to draw upon, and make use of, a wide array of information. We also have to be able to place our experiences and understandings in a wider context, and connect them with our values and commitments. Connoisseurship is something that needs to be worked at—but it is not a technical exercise. The bringing together of the different elements into a whole involves artistry.[9]

Smith places the onus of connoisseurship within the purview of the receivers of cultural ephemera; he does not excuse the institutional purveyors of that same ephemera from the responsibility of contextualizing and presenting "a wide array of information." Indeed, he quotes the art historian and educator Elliot W. Eisner: "Connoisseurship is the art of appreciation. It can be displayed in any realm in which the character, import, or value of objects, situations, and performances is distributed and variable, including educational practice."[10] Here, Eisner seems to be describing connoisseurship and the role of the audience as a performative undertaking; that is, he says, "we" have to be able to contextualize the experience of art-viewing and to artistically create a gestalt from all information provided, perhaps filling in the blank spots as necessary. But when the lights go out, audience gives way to spectatorship. Moreover, Tamara Harvey states in her essay "'What About the Audience?/What About Them?': Spectatorship and Cinematic Pleasure," that connoisseurship

> involves a sense of spectatorial mastery . . . one takes pleasure in being able to recognize and evaluate the differences and similarities which occur between an individual film and the genre as a whole; there is a pleasure in the very sense of familiarity and competence. Moreover, there is also pleasure to be found in the social activity of comparing evaluations of these generic differences with others; discussion and debate over these differences brings out differences and similarities among the viewers.[11]

Connoisseurship, then, might be described as one desired outcome of *any* art form. It is the phenomenon in which literacy grows through the collaborative efforts of curators, makers, and finally audience members and patrons. However, keeping with the dialectic of presenter/institution and audience, screendance audiences, as with any audiences, can react only to what is offered for their consumption by the institution. In other words, the passivity of the audience is assumed: their role is generally to receive the work and value it with their attendance and other methods of support. Thus connoisseurship is limited in scope to the availability of materials institutionally supported or presented for contemplation by audience/ spectators. The audience is not intended to add materially to the intellectual life of the work; a by-product of connoisseurship is that the audience, through post-screening discourse, extends the range of the work beyond the boundaries of the space in which it is sited or transmitted. It is important to note that critics, theorists, and historians are also audience/spectators who, by merging their own practices with elements of spectatorship and connoisseurship, extend the intellectual life of art-works as well.

To return to Tamara Harvey and her titular question, "What about the audience?": what does indeed happen in the dark while the work product of both artists and presenters manifests as projected light onscreen? In the twenty-first century, audience members are preconditioned to function as spectators. Spectatorship is implied, if not assumed, in any postmodern construction having to do with the reading of texts and the semiotic implications of images. Writers of mainstream film and television create scripts that encourage the viewer to share in ironic observations, cynicism, and pop culture referencing, and producers of culture in general often operate on the assumption that their "audience" is given to understanding postmodern techniques of appropriation, which extends to live performance as well. It is safe to assume that an audience, sitting in the dark as screendances are projected before their eyes, will almost involuntarily begin to exercise spectatorial agency, and inherent to spectatorial agency is the impulse to construct meaning from a given set of signs and symbols. Michele Aaron notes that Roland Barthes:

> distinguished between the "writerly" text, in which the reader is productive, and the classical "readerly" text in which "he" merely consumes. For Barthes, the goal of a literary work is "to make the reader no longer a consumer, but a producer of the text." While the reader's role here in interpreting signs—a gesture of agency—is important, the key issue is the general productivity of textual signification. . . . Applying Barthes' ideas to film, textual analysts, through their attention to the many structures of signification . . . would reveal the "galaxy of signifiers" inherent within the film text.[12]

If we accept that Barthes's notion of the "galaxy of signifiers" is manifest as audiences become spectators and apply their collective abilities to the reading of film as text, then the surface quality of the moving image, however seductive, is but a membrane that may be easily breached as one interrogates meaning from the gestalt of the elements present in the film itself. As the signifiers of the film become known, recognized for their literal and or metaphoric values, the audience may be simultaneously enlightened even though they are literally in the dark.

So what then does the audience do with this enlightenment? How do they speak back, if at all, to the institutions that have gathered, packaged, and presented the artwork that is the focus of their programming? As Elliot Eisner writes:

> If connoisseurship is the art of appreciation, criticism is the art of disclosure. Criticism, as Dewey pointed out in *Art as Experience*, has at is end the re-education of perception. . . . The task of the critic is to help us to see. . . . Thus . . . connoisseurship provides criticism with its subject matter. Connoisseurship is private, but criticism is public. Connoisseurs simply need to appreciate what they encounter. Critics, however, must render these qualities vivid by the artful use of critical disclosure . . . effective criticism functions as the midwife to perception. It helps it come into being, then later refines it and helps it to become more acute.[13]

When grafted together, the logical outcome of connoisseurship ("the art of appreciation") and criticism ("the art of disclosure") is a kind of critical connoisseurship that moves beyond matters of taste and style and begins to fulfill Barthes's goal "to make the reader no longer a consumer, but a producer of the text." In this paradigm, the institution and the audience necessarily collaborate in the creation of meaningful cultural moments that resonate beyond the screen and the individual desires of either the institution or the audience.

Because screendance is an interdisciplinary practice that produces cultural products which may be situated in any number of discourses, connoisseurship may serve a larger function to the field of screendance. There is much slippage in the field in regard to formal classification of work that has been re-sited in a new discourse. For instance, it is not uncommon to see a work in the frame of a screendance festival described as an "installation," or to see in the same venue, a live dance performance with video projections. If this work has dance as its provenance, and assumes the histories, practices, knowledges, and received wisdom flowing from dance as such, the connoisseurship that would attach to such an event would likely do so from a similar point of view. Regardless of the subcategories of presentation (installation, etc.), the audience drawn to an event that has framed itself as a *dance on camera* festival (or similar language) will likely be connoisseurs of dance in some manifestation or other. This would seem to be a successful endeavor: to fill a theater with connoisseurs of dance or, by extension, dance on screen. Unfortunately, it may also be critically self-canceling.

As Patrick Phillips points out, audiences are inextricably linked to the institutions that disseminate moving image culture:

> Audiences are seen as constructed by mass-media institutions and exist in a dependent relationship with these institutions. Audiences, especially fans-as-audience, can be seen to be very dependent on the media institutions that produce, promote and sell the product they consume. Just as the spectator can be seen as engaged in a symbiotic (and dependent) relationship with the film text and cinema apparatus, so the audience may be seen as engaged in a similar kind of relationship with the cinema institution.[14]

Yet the nexus between institutions and audiences that Phillips mentions emerges even earlier in the process by which audiences are formed. As connoisseurship is in part an outcome of education in general, we can trace this situation backwards through the mono-disciplinary manner in which students are trained in most academic and conservatory-style higher education programs. Most students who study a particular arts-based curriculum will not, in the end, become professional practitioners of that art (though they may become connoisseurs), institutions of higher education are also educating future audiences of the form. In *The Art Museum as Educator*, a book comprised of case studies focused on the "educational aspect" of museums, the authors note that New York University's "Joint Museum Training Program" with the Metropolitan Museum of Art required courses in connoisseurship as part of their doctorate degree in art history.[15] In the age of postmodernism, connoisseurship has been supplanted by a more relativist point of view; academic and cultural institutions continue to act as agents of both education and connoisseurship while they function as conduits to content produced by artists, scholars, and arbiters of value based on those choices.

In recent years, screendance has entered academia in the form of courses that focus on videodance or technologically mediated dance. Yet, however positive this recognition of screendance may be, course materials and teaching methodologies vary greatly from institution to institution. There is as yet no definitive canon (and in keeping with postmodern notions of porosity and polyvocality, perhaps we should think of a canon as ever-evolving) from which one may draw either factual references or artistic interpretations. Hence, the dissemination of information and the availability of screening materials are largely a product of the teacher's access to the international screendance community and its creative output—a by-product of connoisseurship. Often, courses are undertaken with limited resources and reflect a lack of specificity regarding the placement of screendance within a larger framework of the history of dance, video art, cinema, the visual arts, and media in general. As a consequence of the difficulty in obtaining a cohesive body of films for screening in courses, work in the genre that is readily available or easily accessible becomes exemplary of the field as well as a sort of default history. Meanwhile, the appropriate scholarship related to that material, as well as the contextualization, critique, and framing of it, are often nonexistent or inadequate. Furthermore, as most screendance courses (in the United States especially) grow out of preexisting dance programs, whose mission it is to articulate their course work through the lens of dance practice, the analysis of work used for reference as well as in-class, student-produced projects are generally presented and critiqued through the formal structures of choreography and performance. Although objectivity is a preferred methodology in academia, due to the lack of a screendance canon and related literature, there is a considerable amount of subjectivity involved in the institutionalization of screendance—a further example of the production of knowledge based on connoisseurship.

Screendance is situated in the folds of postmodernism, yet with no fixed set of tools typifying or denoting the provenance of screendance, its materiality oscillates between technologies of representation found in *either* modern or postmodern art-making strategies. However, the modernist desires of dance and film create a palpable tension with the postmodern desires of digital culture, which is often the endpoint of screendance both materially and strategically. This tension, along with the competing desires of the audience (the desires for narrative structure or not, for real bodies or not), creates a schism that leaves screendance in theoretical limbo, unlike other areas of art practice with more clearly defined foci. In the 1980s, for example, painting was, according to the critic Barbara Rose, an art form united enough on a "sufficient number of critical issues" so that it was possible to isolate those issues that bound the "serious painters" together as a group.[16] Rose stated that the painter's recognizable esthetic "defines itself in conscious opposition to photography and all forms of mechanical reproduction which seek to deprive the art work of its unique 'aura.'"[17] The "serious painters" Rose alludes to were able to identify the opposition due in large part to the plethora of curatorial activism and critical writing in the era by a new breed of critic—among them Douglas Crimp, who organized the exhibition called *Pictures* at Artists Space in New York City in the fall of 1977. Crimp wrote of the exhibition:

> In choosing the word pictures for this show, I hoped to convey not only the work's most salient characteristic—recognizable images—but also and importantly the ambiguities it sustains. As is typical of what has come to be called postmodernism, this new work is not confined to any particular medium; instead, it makes use of photography, film, performance, as well as traditional modes of painting, drawing, and sculpture. Picture, used colloquially, is also nonspecific: a picture book might be a book of drawings or photographs, and in common speech a painting, drawing, or print is often called, simply, a picture. Equally important for my purposes, picture, in its verb form, can refer to a mental process as well as the production of an aesthetic object.[18]

Both Crimp and Barbara Rose thus take an activist role in championing their vision for art: Rose with a manifesto-like text for the catalog of *American Painting: The Eighties*, the exhibition which she organized at the Grey Art Gallery at New York University in 1980; and Crimp in *Pictures*. Both make their claims and interrogations based not only on the facts in evidence in their respective areas of interest but also by simultaneously adopting a posture of connoisseurship, relying as well on their passion and *gut reaction* to the work in question. In the case of Rose, the modernist critic, connoisseurship may seem apropos, but Crimp is the postmodernist, an important critic in the development of that theory, particularly in the area of photography, whom one might surmise would adhere to a more relativist approach to criticism. Nonetheless, Crimp allows for the co-existence of connoisseurship and postmodernism in his essay, *The Photographic Activity of Postmodernism*.[19] He calls on the connoisseurship of the "old fashioned art historian" to assist in proving the relative value of photography, in order to make a case for its inclusion in and competition for the "wall space of the museum." And while connoisseurship may seem antithetical to the very nature of postmodernism, Crimp states, "What interests me is the subjectivization of photography, the ways in which the connoisseurship of the photograph's 'spark of chance' is converted into a connoisseurship of the photograph's style."[20] Crimp reinforces the notion that at the heart of every picture is the hand of the artist, that one can detect stylistic difference from image to image and that it is the hand of the artist that undermines and subverts art history itself. Crimp, the postmodern critic, arrives through the rigorous processing of visual and textual data at the conclusion that style, the most subjective trait, is still of value in understanding and reckoning with the work of art in the postmodern era. In other words, connoisseurship is not *the* tool but rather *one* tool in the postmodern critic's toolkit. And for both Crimp and Rose, the catalog essays and the exhibitions illuminate each other and add a level of significance to their connoisseurship that might, in the presence of only the artworks organized for their exhibitions (or only the texts), diminish their individual efforts.

A primary function of connoisseurship then, is to illuminate and articulate difference and provenance. As screendance begins to claim more territory outside its own borders and venture into the domains of other practices (film, video art, installation art), the body of knowledge necessary to contextualize and frame a conversation about the various forms of hybridity at work expands exponentially. If a consequence of screendance's territorial expansion is the appropriation of already theorized discrete practices, then that appropriation must necessarily include the extant theoretical and historical discourses attached to the appropriated practices. This is the domain of connoisseurship: the active pursuit of knowledges that situate and honor an art form, and enable ways of bridging those knowledges through equally active discourses and reportage.

Screendance festivals now routinely include "installation" work in their programming. Often billed even more specifically as "site specific installations," the institutions do not tend to offer much substantive rationale for what constitutes site-specificity or how the work in question is in fact a part of the larger discourse on installation art in general.[21] The appropriation of art-world terminology without the attendant art-world theory leaves the viewer only half-full. If connoisseurship is to lead to an advanced literacy in the field, then institutions need to do more than simply appropriate form. Installation of moving-image material has been deeply theorized in the art world. Take, for example, Kate Mondloch's exposition on spectatorship as it relates to the discourse surrounding installation art:

> Contemporary art practice and criticism, profoundly influenced by Marxist critiques of alienation, phenomenological critiques of Cartesianism, and post-structuralist critiques of authorship, conventionally understands the spectator's active participation to be progressive for purportedly engendering an empowered, critically aware viewing subject. . . . In sum, the critical discourse surrounding this art form pits active, open-ended reception (especially associated with Brecht's materialist and collectivist notion of aesthetic reception) against passive consumption.[22]

The "spectator's active participation" to which Mondloch refers is not only limited to installation art, but marks postmodernism in general. It extends to all areas of critical response emanating from the event, object, or situation, and it is a driving force in the idea that meaning as it pertains to art is no longer fixed but rather a fluid and flexible construct. In order to participate in this fluid construction of meaning, all parties, including organizers, presenters, institutions, and the academy must necessarily be activists, informed and *informing* consumers and disseminators of cultural production.

As screendance becomes institutionalized, the process by which a canon and/or a set of critical criteria and esthetic strategies for assessing the field is built by trial and error, consensus, and curatorial activism. Both academia and festivals as well as more independent efforts to disseminate the culture of screendance are built on a foundation of decisions about the relative value of individual works of screendance and the myriad histories and narratives of the field. These decisions are subjective and personal, whether by committee or individual vision. Thus, the development of an informed and educated connoisseurship that recognizes and values plurality and postmodern theoretical discourse benefits both makers of screendance and audiences as well.

Again, the screen is a space of competing desires, and screendance as a practice reflects a similar dialectic. On the one hand, screendance exhibits a desire for virtuosic dance encapsulated within a screenic frame; on the other, a competing desire for the practice to dislodge itself from its tethers to traditional representations of dance and its tendency to conform to the entertainment value of cinema. What deepens these proposals and extrapolates the desire from each "act of engagement" between artist and media, between audience and artist or critic and film, is discourse; or as the art writer Michael Brenson calls it, *conversation*. He writes:

> Conversation is fundamental. It is part of the machinery of culture, of society, of the self. . . . It stretches the imagination and makes it possible to envisage new narratives at the end of a century in which some of the most controlling master narratives have collapsed . . . to converse [is] to be exposed.[23]

The kind of conversation that Brenson describes can come only from a deeply engaged connoisseurship, one in which all factions of the "machinery of culture" collaborate. In screendance, that means jostling the status quo: granting agency to performers, taking curatorial risks, giving voice to important cultural moments in a field that has typically opted out of the kind of critical discourse that allows, and encourages a field to expand

and grow. Perhaps a more adventurous engagement between dance and its mediated image might allow for its hybridity and experimental nature to push the field toward the unknown, toward new kinds of "acts of engagement" that may deepen and amplify screendance for both audiences and artists alike.

When connoisseurship succeeds in amplifying the resonance of screendance—that is to say, when the transmission of the culture of bodies on screen transcends form—then indeed, seeing is forgetting the name of the thing one sees: critical connoisseurship presents the possibility of naming it again.

CHAPTER 9

Toward a Theory of Screendance

Screendance has been frozen in a period of adolescence for an extraordinarily long time. It is a field that is, in a way, balkanized into communities that are constantly rediscovering ontologies and phenomenologies of the practice as if for the first time. Festivals, publications, and periodicals that comment on or exhibit such work encourage this eternal adolescence by reinforcing a kind of entrenched status quo. It may be that artists, in the moment of creation, are fully engaged with and committed to situating their work in tributaries that flow from fully realized movements with historically diverse theoretical concerns. However, as that work leaves the cradle of its maker and circulates throughout the communities of viewership and critical analysis that attach to screendance, the gap between the maker's desires and the often-competing desires of art and entertainment widens. The twin trends of festival screenings and streaming video sites tend to operate within social spaces that avoid critical analysis, and as such have helped to defer the possibilities of an emergence from prolonged adolescence into "adulthood," as well as the kind of deep reflection that comes with such an evolution.[1]

Throughout this book I have proposed a number of approaches to the field of screendance, with the aim of raising the level of critical discourse and encouraging a deepening of the practice. In the preceding pages, I have suggested activist curating, connoisseurship through close reading, and critical analysis of work in the field, a flexible and porous historical continuum, and the excavation of genres to identify patterns and trends in screendance as means of scaffolding a theory of screendance. This chapter demonstrates methodologies for viewing, discussing, and making works, by implementing and performing these paradigms, and herein models and theorizes the ways in which such paradigms may be put into practice for the purpose of creating historical linkages, broadening the culture of screendance, and tethering screendance to discourses in the visual arts, cinema, and contemporary theory.

Screendance is simultaneously conformative and performative. It *conforms* to the materiality of its host while *performing* its desired identity; dance framed by and situated within the architecture of camera space and its attendant production technologies molds to those devices and their inherent boundaries. It does so while simultaneously attempting to maintain its recognizable danceness. Even so, screendance culture is an expanded culture, a site-specific practice that, if true to form, moves beyond the simple migration of dance from the stage (with the inherent motivations and logic of dance intact) and re-sites bodies in motion in a filmic or screenic space. Such spaces have specificity that is often at odds with choreographic logic, which has been conceptualized in *actual* three-dimensional space. Screenic, cinematic, or filmic spaces are two-dimensional spaces, *illusionary* spaces, and as such are spaces of secondary witnessing. While viewing a screendance it is clear that bodies *were* in motion in some prior temporal moment, and that those same bodies *did* perform in real space in real time. But those phenomena are in the past in a dimensional, temporal space, one that is not the present and not where we sit. The audience is thus composed of secondary witnesses to the kinesthetic and performative moments that have been recast in screenic space, which is nevertheless still hosted by the bodies that were inscribed upon and which, in turn, inscribed the method of recording. The bodies that we view on screen are also illusions. We, the viewers, repatriate them to the locales, sites, and venues in which they appear to be "performing" and simultaneously project histories and other narratives upon those bodies. This book suggests a break with dance-centric narratives of both provenance (the histories of screendance) and reading (the surfaces of screendance) in order to crack open the discourse around the field and force it out of its prolonged adolescence. The model of exhaustion that Andre Lepecki has proposed about dance in general (and about which we read in chapter 7) ironically extends to screendance even in its still nascent stage: it has been institutionalized prior to the maturation of the field, eternally youthful and critically unformed.[2]

Through its own kind of locative devices such as visual language, exhibition venues, and marginalized discourse, screendance has historically positioned itself apart from the larger art world. Attempts by scholars or others to intellectualize screendance or to tether it to histories and practices beyond than those that are dance-centric (film being a notable exception), have largely been ignored. But this clearly denies the way in which discourses about art are inevitably tied to critical masses of similarly inclined artists and thinkers. When thinking about art in the broadest sense, movements, schools of practice, periods, and styles come to mind, and each such delineation alludes to a particular critical moment. For instance, Abstract Expressionism recalls Clement Greenberg, Harold Rosenberg, and the larger framework of Modernism. Postmodern practices such as video and performance art engage philosophers like Derrida, Foucault, and Benjamin. By contrast, when we think about dance (whose subcategories might include ballet, modern, postmodern, jazz, and tap), there is less language available by which to frame the field in larger propositions regarding critical moments. The delineations we find in the field of dance, as opposed to those suggested for visual arts, tend to be about style and technique rather than larger theoretical constructs, though they do inform viewing practices and create context. When we articulate the next level of identity, that of choreographic specificity—for instance, the work of Martha Graham, Merce Cunningham, or Trisha Brown—we invoke another set of semiotic references and resonant images embedded in both the practice of technique and the techniques of individual authorship: the traits of difference. We seek recognizable traits of authorship as well as genre specificity from our modern dance, traits that not only separate the techniques from other techniques but also separate a work's esthetics from that of other choreographers. Screendance expands the culture of dance and necessarily demands a similarly expanded notion of theory in general in order to support its own weight.

One strategy for such an expanded theory of screendance involves placing the practice in preexisting, recognizable discourses applicable to the field. Throughout this text, I have used the terms modernist (or modernism) and/or postmodern to frame discussions about various artistic undertakings. Both Noël Carroll and Sally Banes stated that modernism in the Greenbergian analysis is about the purity of form: "the Modernist enterprise is committed to purity. Under the modernist dispensation, each art form is beholden to its constitutive medium. It is the project of each art form to explore, foreground and acknowledge its own nature."[3] This description of the proprieties of modernism would seem to either exclude or catalog a particular approach to screendance. The idea, embedded in the modernist proposal, that each art form represented is indebted to its own nature (the idea of "purity" of form) not only precludes the intermingling of contemporary forms of representation and expression but ossifies the forms that already exist and permanently fixes their boundaries.

Regarding postmodernism, the critic Arthur Danto has noted that "Postmodernism, an authentic style which has emerged within the post-historical period was generally and defiantly characterized by an indifference to the kind of purity Greenberg saw as the goal of an historical development."[4] Although the two eras overlap considerably and even co-exist (however uncomfortably) for a time, Danto's quote coupled with that of Banes and Carroll offer antagonistic landmarks by which we can triangulate the territory in which screendance has sought to co-exist among the other art forms during succeeding eras. These markers and linguistic constructions seem essential to my theory.

History provides us with a foundation for articulating ideas about art and culture. Art in general aligns itself with numerous categories and subcategories, offering infinite combinations of intertextuality, and is immediately knowable by its contextualization within art-historical referencing systems. For example, "a painter in the cubist style," "a sculptor in the realist style," "a performance in the futurist style," or even "a futurist/realist/postmodern appropriation of a Dada-like collage" are all fairly common ways to articulate hybrid practices. These descriptions bring to mind works of art with gravitas and depth of history, and also contain semiotic resonance. They furthermore conjure works that are tethered to distinct historical moments that inform both the maker and the viewer about process, substance, materiality, and content. They also inform the critic, historian, or scholar and an ongoing dialog is perhaps most important in the sustainability of any practice. Without the participation of the third party, whose job it is to inscribe a cultural reference to the work of art, the circle is incomplete. Art feeds on the external world and also on itself. It is a conversation that happens on many levels simultaneously: the maker, the viewer, the translator, the gallerist, the presenter, the consumer, and the reporter, together create a feedback loop that has no beginning and no end but is a kind of persistent present. These infinite loops are often initiated through the visual culture of an exhibition.

In the art world proper, a curated exhibition would generally not include Abstract Expressionist paintings along with religious iconography, nor would neorealist paintings be grouped with color field paintings, unless the curatorial thesis were to make a point about difference. Yet, in screendance, especially in festival settings, there is no delineation between comedic dance films and site-specific dance films, or narrative and non-narrative work, or solo expressionistic dance films and intergenerational work. In other words, we have not made the effort to parse screendance into contextual frames of reference as other art forms have done. And while screendance it is more difficult to identify or delineate movements or genres (much less to locate identifiable authorship separate from choreographic identity), this lack of self-definition is cause for concern in a field that already teeters on marginality. Though the end point of such work is a *media construction,* equal parts moving-image production and dance, screendance is largely perceived as a production of the dance world. As such, it is sheltered from the discourse that surrounds the history and production of either film or video, and instead is often seen as at most an extension of dance—it perhaps moves dance into a new venue, but is still, in the end, seen as a product *of* dance. Thus, despite screendance's hybrid form, it has been moving forward without the benefit of a critical mass of theory by which to inform a discourse that would raise the level of understanding and production to that of the other arts. This diminishes not just the value of screendance work in a historical continuum but also the viewing of the work in that it is largely presented in a decontextualized setting. Creating frames of reference and prisms through which a work of art is viewed enables the work of art by inserting it into an ongoing dialog with other work. Perhaps more importantly, it encourages the kind of metaphor, allusion, and intertextual referencing that is crucial to art in general.

The Australian dance artists Richard James Allen and Karen Pearlman propose that screendance can be defined as "stories told by the body."[5] Their term implies that the corporeal body is present in the work and that the body is the instrument of inscription, much as a pen on paper articulates other languages. It suggests that the body is the center of the work, the focus, even as the body is writing simultaneously a kind of personal history or diary. "Stories told by the body" through the medium of film or video are compelling and altogether distinct from the experience of concert dance yet the term implies a sense of narrative within the screendance. Perhaps amending "stories told by the body" to include stories "not told by the body" is a more accurate representation of the desires of the field. For Allen and Pearlman, the filmmaker creates a work from the common language of dancing bodies. As the lingua franca of dancing bodies, bodies in motion, or bodies in repose is by itself deeply poetic and highly metaphoric, it is the filmmakers' responsibility to recorporealize the fragmented and disjointed bits of dance captured on film or in digital media into a cohesive whole: it is not necessarily appropriate to force that collected imagery to "tell a story." To use the metaphor of painting, there is room for the equivalent of both impressionist and color field pictures in the practice of screendance, but, again, there is a need for the independent articulation of each in order to build a critical mass of knowledges in the field.

The art of filmmaking translates the corporeal liveness of dance in its indigenous form to the often-deadening space of the screen. In the space between the choreographer's and the filmmaker's eye, the synergistic relationship between dance and the moving image is articulated. Such synergy produces a work for the screen that operates on a visceral, kinesthetic plane as well as on a logical, narrative, or abstract one. The camera, however, consumes all that enters its frame: it is omnivorous. The body in motion or in action contextualizes the work, but it is the implicitly carnal, predatory nature of the camera that enlivens the dance as it plays out on screen. The philosopher Merleau-Ponty suggests that an action of the body produces a synergistic sense of itself that is at once both internal and external.[6] To those who experience the body in motion, the dancing body becomes known visually (or tactilely) as simultaneously it becomes known to itself. The act of moving in space transmits information both outward and inward at the same instant. What an audience perceives as it witnesses the dancer dance is a kind of performative, autobiographical writing—writing in real, spatial, dimensional time. The audience perceives movement (dance) as the body gains insight into itself, as it inscribes its narrative in an ephemeral social space. Creating a film from that ephemeral body-writing is a way of not only extending the metaphors of dancing bodies but also of producing an infinitely viewable cultural artifact.

John Martin offers a mode for understanding the phenomenology of the transmission of kinesthetic awareness (see chap. 3). According to the dance historian Susan Manning, "Martin theorized what he called 'metakinesis' to describe the "process whereby the spectator reexperienced 'the physical and the psychical' dimensions of dance movement," the situation in which the viewer is drawn into the dance.[7] This is what Walter Benjamin has referred to as the aura; and in screendance, the recovery of the aura makes tangible what is, in Martin's proposal, intangible. Much has been written about the way in which we, the viewers, embody a kind of sympathetic response to live dancing bodies; relatively less has been written about how that sympathetic, kinesthetic sensation is translated to the screen.[8] This challenge also extends to the viewer, who must forego preconceived ideas about dance in order to fully embody the experience of viewing screendance.

Ultimately, though, in the production of media, the director's eye defines what we see—through framing, camera position, and other aspects of cinematography practice. Screendance has a tendency to be viewed or programmed as a choreographer's medium, and it is often the choreographer who is foregrounded as the dominant force within the work. It is also true that film is historically a *directed* medium; perhaps therein lies the basis for this definitional tension. Choreography is not at odds with screendance by any means, but at the risk of restating, screendance is ultimately a moving-image inscription of numerous visual elements, among them dancing bodies. A "directed" film is one in which there is an objective distance between the dance and the cinematic articulation of it. The director's work is in the details of bringing a dance to life on screen; this process begins in the composition of moving images as the dance is mined for its cinematic possibilities. The director works in much the same way as an archeologist might: unearthing, revealing, and ultimately reconnecting the disparate parts collected at the site of the excavation. As the process unfolds, the dance becomes its filmic self. Often, the movement the choreographer invented *in studio* bends to a new shape and in a sense, choreographic ego gives way to the emergent identity of the film. Somewhere within the social space of a film shoot, the *work* reveals itself. It may be in the shooting, it may be in editing; but it requires openness to the possibilities of the medium to carve or compel its own form.

Although screendance is a collaborative art, there is *one* privileged point of view in the making of a film. It is through the camera's lens that screendance is built, shot by shot, frame by frame. This method of construction is further articulated in the editing process. But the accretion of danced moments as they are unearthed and cataloged, archived and arranged, is the territory of the director. And while the choreographer and director may be the same person, a set of outside eyes, an alternative esthetic, and a preexisting relationship with the medium of film or video can often unearth something nascent or germinal in the dance. Far from closing down screendance, this fact suggests that it is the screendance director's central challenge to grasp Merleau-Ponty's ideas about kinesthetic sensation and Martin's "metakinesis," and to both migrate and translate those concepts to the frame, thereby extending the metaphors of dance into a new *filmic* space. In that transition from "live" to screen, screendance then redefines and questions the language of dance while also interrogating the nature of the moving image and its relationship to dance. In short, the transition from live to screen moves toward an ineffable gestalt in which the whole is not only greater than the sum of its parts, but the parts are also transformed in the process.

The act of making a screendance often becomes ritualistic given the deep focus the situation of production requires. It is often quiet in the space of production, and if the production is small, perhaps only a dancer/ choreographer and a cameraperson, the tendency to become hyperfocused invites a kind of ritualistic performance. In this space, where a performance that is only ever known to those present at that time and place, the camera becomes a witness, even an intimate of the body, and as that witness defines the activity in the production space. Such is the power of cameras to define events both culturally and actually. When a camera is brought into an already unfolding event, we know that the nature of that event is inexorably changed.

That is to say, in the presence of the camera, dance often becomes less kinesthetic and more concerned with nuance, minutiae, and a kind of exploration of tactility and surface. The ritual of production often manifests itself as a kind of self-imposed slow motion, in which the dancer enters a state of self-awareness catalyzed by the camera's presence. This translates to the visual equivalent of a meditation on movement itself, often conflicting with the kinesthetic possibilities of the space of the screen. The camera exerts a force that slows time, even breath, resulting in a hyper-awareness on the part of its subject. The irony in this phenomenon is that the camera is able to capture events and motion invisible to the eye and, postproduction provides numerous tools for slowing time. It is possible that the altered sense of temporality in the space of screendance comes from a culturally embedded relationship to cameras, which implies that motionlessness is a prerequisite for creating a photograph: one must pose for the camera. In the creation of a screendance, the dancer's *limited* motion becomes a kind of tacit assumption that the camera operator will then *create* motion via cinematic techniques. It is another irony that in this scenario, the camera operator, by default, becomes a choreographer, or at least "choreographs" the camera's trajectory through space while the dancer's kinesthetic voice is often muted either by choice or by default.

In the earliest days of video art, cameras were often brought into the artistic workplace to record deeply personal, private, and often ritualistic performances. These performances for the camera were less about entertainment and more about catalyzing a profound personal exploration of psychic space and embodied experience. The camera, as witness, acted as shamanistic guide, electronically "writing" the piece as it unfolded and thus exerting a kind of agency that both enabled and disabled the performance taking place before it. The camera enabled the performance inasmuch as it functioned as an ersatz audience, a silent and nonjudgmental audience. It disabled the performance in that the resulting videotape could never be anything other than a simulation. It was always only a referent to the original.

The camera focuses the act of seeing in a way that is quite different than the perceptual act that one might practice as a matter of habit. Camera-looking is an active performance that frames an event and elevates it while "screening out" all other information. It implies a reverence for that which is framed and eschews all that is outside the frame. In doing so, it parses activity into essential and nonessential, absent and present, and presupposes the editing process, which further parses individual moments of mediated performance into even smaller partitions. One might suppose that the mediation of live dance by a recording device would distance the viewer from the activity framed, but it is the opposite that occurs for the cameraperson as she engages the dancer within the frame. The phenomenon is one in which the camera becomes a prosthetic for seeing and transforms the ordinary into the extraordinary. Through this vision-prosthetic, a new kind of intimacy is created between the camera operator and the performer. However, intimacy in the space of mediated representation is conceptually fraught.

In the history of art since the twentieth century, mediated images of bodies, especially female bodies, have been both theorized and fetishized. Images that circulate via media are contextualized by the literacy particular to the media in which they are inscribed, since mediation not only frames its subject matter in the formal sense but also "frames" the discourse around its subject. In the case of screendance, the potential of the camera to heighten intimacy (with the performer) is also the potential to instantiate desire and sexualize its subject. In her seminal essay *Visual Pleasure and Narrative Cinema* (1975), the feminist film theorist Laura Mulvey entered

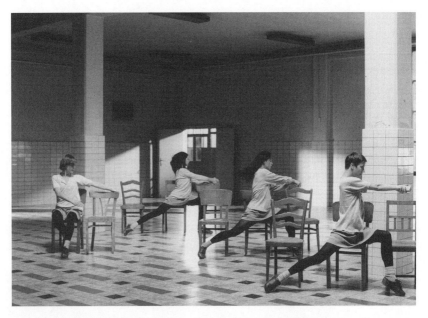

Figure 9.1: *Rosas Danst Rosas* (1997), Anne Teresa De Keersmaeker
photographer (c) Herman Sorgeloos, courtesy Anne Teresa De Keersmaeker

into popular and critical culture the notion of the "male gaze." Mulvey proposed that the conditions of cinema, including viewing spaces, historical confluences, and demographics (who is viewing, etc.), facilitate both voyeurism and objectification of female characters in cinema. She linked her notions of fetishism to Freud and Marx in implicating the male viewer and his participation in the fetishizing of female bodies on screen. In the essay Mulvey argues that a radical shift away from the presentation of women as passive objects of male desire is necessary (in mainstream cinema, especially as produced by Hollywood) in order to liberate women from the oppressiveness and manipulations of the male gaze. She states:

> Woman displayed as sexual object is the leit-motif of erotic spectacle: from pin-ups to striptease, from Ziegfeld to Busby Berkeley, she holds the look, plays to and signifies male desire. Mainstream film neatly combined spectacle and narrative. (Note, however, how the musical song-and-dance numbers break the flow of the diegesis.) The presence of woman is an indispensable element of spectacle in normal narrative film, yet her visual presence tends to work against the development of a story line, to freeze the flow of action in moments of erotic contemplation.[9]

Mulvey notes how, historically, women's sexuality has been foregrounded in both theater and film (specifically noting the films of Busby Berkeley). This observation bears disproportionately on screendance, as the camera exacerbates and elevates that which may be most easily objectified through its own aggressive performance. However, cameras do not self-select framing, depth of field, or close-up. Those choices are made by directors, and as such the responsibility for such "erotic spectacles" is the purview of the makers of screendance. Mulvey further suggests that privileging the (female's) esthetic qualities of beauty, sensuality, and so forth leads to a situation that "freezes the look, fixates the spectator and prevents him from achieving any distance from the image in front of him."[10]

While Mulvey's essay does not explicitly address screendance, it does provide a provocative template that may be appropriated to address issues particular to the genre. Mulvey often speaks of the apparatus of the moving image, and her observations in "Visual Pleasure" and other texts may be adapted to theorize screendance. For example, in her later book from 1996, *Fetishism and Curiosity*, Mulvey explains, from a Marxist point of view, that "a commodity's market success depends on the erasure of the marks of production," allowing commodity fetishism to "triumph as spectacle." This is an apt description for the shift from experimental screendance works made in the 1960s and '70s, such as Merce Cunningham and Charles Atlas's *Blue Studio*, to the more highly produced and cinematic or televisual works currently encountered in festivals and broadcast television. Such films (for instance, Wim Wenders' 3D film *Pina*, director Thierry De Mey's rework of William Forsythe's *One Flat Thing, Reproduced*, or Mike Figgis' *The Co(te)lette Film, a rework of* Dutch choreographer Ann Van den Broek's dance for the stage) follow the model of European and Canadian dance films of the late 1980s and '90s, and continue to dominate the international festival circuit. Though previously shot on 16 or 35 mm film, now often produced in high definition video, their lush surface quality, combined with sensual choreography performed by stunningly talented and appealing dancers, altered the landscape of screendance. In moving away from a style of production in which the maker's marks were clearly in evidence, dance films by DV8, La La La Human Steps, L'Esquisse, Phillipe Decoufle, and others effaced the "marks of production" found in work flowing from video art or experimental film, in favor of a style that allowed for more mainstream distribution. Often highly produced and moving toward spectacle, this work at times perpetuates Mulvey's notion of the male gaze in its often-sexualized depictions of women. This is evident even in work created *by* women, such as the Belgian choreographer and director Anne Teresa De Keersmaeker. In numerous dance films by De Keersmaeker, including *Achterland* and *Rosas Danst Rosas*, the camera invades the very private spaces of her dancer's bodies, uncovering or exploiting moments in which the vulnerability of the (female) dancer is transposed to a highly sexualized screen image. The "charge" of these screen images is enabled and amplified by the privilege of the camera to negotiate personal space and extrapolate sexuality from moments that on stage would be fleeting and possibly insignificant. However, the performance of the camera is perhaps underacknowledged as an element in the subsequent reading of screendance. Peggy Phelan states that "the camera's own performativity needs to be read as theater."[11] As the camera frames an originally live, performed event, it also adds a layer of editorialization and even commentary to that event.

A close viewing of two well-known screendance works may help to illuminate how the camera exacerbates intimacy, and at times exploits it. *Rosas Danst Rosas* (1997) (De Keersmaeker and Thierry De Mey), though a compelling and seductively beautiful film, is one in which the camera exercises an almost predatory presence. The film is made up of a number of scenes; in one, four women seated on mismatched chairs in a large tiled room begin a gestural, rhythmic phrase accompanied by Thierry De Mey's original score. Following the initial close-up of one dancer prone across three chairs, the film cuts to a wide shot of the four women. The combination of De Mey's pulsing score and the performance of repetitious choreographic phrases builds toward an inevitable change, which comes in the form of a cut to the camera in motion, circling, stalking, seemingly watching unseen as the all-woman cast repeats gestural sets of movement, and the camera eye moves with the implication of voyeurism. Coupled with the dancers' sense of their own bodies, the rhythmic expelling of breath, and the mesmerizing, repetitious score, *Rosas Danst Rosas* feels ominous and foreboding, as if we are waiting for the kettle to boil over. The relief comes in the cut from the circling camera to the close-ups of individual dancers shot from the chest up. The cuts come quicker, and the bodies are fragmented into their parts: a hand grabs wrist, two hands smooth hair, eyes make contact with the camera, a hand darts between thighs, a dancer fleetingly cups her breast in her hand. The camera picks up these small gestures and amplifies them. The viewer becomes aware of the dancers' constant touching of their own bodies in ways that, while not overtly sexual, become over time sexualized by the accretion of visual cues coming from both the choreography and the production of it for screen. There is a kind of evanescent flirtation between dancer and camera that pervades *Rosa Danst Rosas*; the camera, through its own choreography, seems anthropomorphized, restlessly changing positions as a viewer might, to better see the dancers.

The treatment of female bodies in De Keersmaeker and De Mey's film has historical precedent. In "The Kinesthetics of Avant-Garde Dance Film: Deren and Harris," Amy Greenfield offers a virtually frame-by-frame recounting of Harris's often screened and cited dance film *Nine Variations on a Dance Theme* (1967) performed by Bettie de Jong.[12] Though the film is often noted as seminal to the field, there is very little actual writing on it and what there is, is mostly written as a formalist, descriptive, often slightly mythologized anti-critique. Boston's WGBH Television, which holds a video master, notes that, "This film work was acquired by WGBH for inclusion in the series *Artists on Artists*, which was broadcast as part of *Artist's Showcase*. The synopsis states:

> A female dancer repeats a short dance theme nine times to a soundtrack of piano and flute. As she performs the theme, the dancer is shot from different angles to yield nine variations. The first variations are composed of longer shots that capture the body and movements of the dancer in full. These variations are accompanied by a soundtrack of slow-tempo piano. The later variations are composed of many shorter shots that capture the components of the dancer's body and movements. These variations are accompanied by an increasingly up-tempo soundtrack of piano and flute.[13]

By way of contrast, Greenfield's more lengthy account offers a multitude of detail and formal observations that, while imminently useful, ignores the more troubling aspects of the work itself. What Greenfield describes as "making love through the camera with the movement"[14]—an idea that she attributes to Harris yet shares herself—might also be read as an extreme act of violence perpetrated by the camera's invasiveness and the evolution of Harris's nine variations over the course of the film. Though rendered somewhat less violent in its invasion of the dancer's personal space thanks to the historical distance of the piece, a viewing of the film in the present still demonstrates the camera's carnal appetite.[15]

Greenfield begins with a description of the first movement of the piece, the theme upon which the next eight variations are based:

> In Harris's 12-minute, black-and-white 16 mm short, Bettie de Jong lies on her side in the middle of a large, sunny loft, with a wall of windows behind her. She starts to move, circling her arm in an act of discovery of space. She contracts, spirals up to her knees, continues to turn until she stands and lifts her leg and arms. Turning, spiraling in plie, she returns to floor and the same position in which she started. No one movement is separate, and the whole phrase is structured as a constant speed loop.[16]

Greenfield's recounting of Harris's *Nine Variations* continues a movement-by-movement analysis of the form of the film relying on highly descriptive, formal observations, such as issues of "free kinesthetic flow", dynamics, and continuity. She moves beyond a strictly formal analysis of Harris's film and begins to ascribe anthropomorphic qualities to the production of meaning in the work, and also to the camera and the filmmaking apparatus itself. After describing the seventh variation, for example, Greenfield writes: "In the eighth variation, we fully experience Harris's own sensation of making love to the dancer with the camera. The camera, in extreme close-up, seems to be inside her. Outer body and inner sensation are conflated."[17] In her positive and admittedly reverent analysis of Harris's work, Greenfield nevertheless articulates a model in which the clearly male-identified object of inscription, the camera and its probing lens, crosses the boundary from objective witness to carnal predator. In the eighth variation, Harris's camera not only fragments de Jong's body as Greenfield alludes to, but invades her sex. Clearly, the cuts from "hand to foot to knee, to a lock of hair" that Greenfield describes have a very different charge and implied meaning than those in which the camera lingers on the *V* of de Jong's pubic area or the roundness of her buttocks penetrating the tightly focused frame as she circles to the floor. Cutting from de Jong on her back, legs parting to open her crotch to the tautness of fabric over breasts, the film cuts back to crotch as we see the dancer then in full frame, arms spread wide, legs open, body prone. Certainly this may be read as sensual, as Greenfield implies, but such a reading also implies a number of other conditions. The viewer has no knowledge of the dancer's agency in *Nine Variations*, whether she indeed wished for or consented to the filmmakers desire "to make love" to her "through the camera," or if the camera and ultimately the film simply consumed her corporeality and elided her agency in the process. Screendance does perform a desire for a new kind of body, the "cinematic body" that Greenfield describes. Nonetheless, in *Nine Variations*, what we witness is a violated body.

Comparing *Nine Variations* to Maya Deren's *A Study in Choreography for Camera* with Talley Beatty, Greenfield states: "Harris here extends Deren's concept of overlapping cuts to symphonic proportions, a musical climax communicating human transcendence through dance, turning the mortal, finite body into an organism of infinite possibility." In the end, the "cinematic body" is in this case an objectified body, upon which are projected the fantasies of the filmmaker and the semiotics inherent in the screenic representation of de Jong's sexualized, fetishized corpus. While there are similarities between Deren's *A Study in Choreography for Camera*, which Greenfield uses as counterpoint to *Nine Variations*, there are significant differences as well. *Nine Variations,* though a silent film per se, has a score layered over the film that greatly enhances and amplifies the "symphonic proportions" of the film. The body in *Nine Variations* is tethered, confined in a room that has no external reference other than the shimmering light of day visible from the windows. Her body is cut off from the natural world, and there are no signs of habitation present in the room. Given the starkness of the space, it could be a prison or a chic loft; there is no way to tell. In Deren's *A Study in Choreography for Camera*, on the other hand, the film is silent and there is no overlaid score that artificially enhances the performance or the editing. The dancer's body (Beatty), is also fragmented by the camera's framing and editing, but he moves freely from interior to exterior spaces, ultimately seen against the landscape, implying a kind of human transcendence that is quite different than that which Greenfield describes as in evidence in *Nine Variations*. At the end of *A Study in Choreography for Camera*, Beatty transcends gravity and time, the natural laws, as Deren creates her version of the cinematic body through editing. At the end of *Nine Variations*, Greenfield observes, "The most personal shots in the film are the final ones: de Jong's face as she looks with longing toward the floor, as if it were her lover to whom she is returning, until her cheek comes to rest gently on the floor and the camera comes with her to its final rest."[18] Contrary to Greenfield's positive reading of *Nine Variations*, which emphasizes the "transforming [of] the body," the film in fact inscribes the kind of cinematic violence and carnal desire that Laura Mulvey addresses in her "Visual Pleasure and Narrative Cinema" article. The female body in *Nine Variations* is fetishized by the synesthesia of camera, music, location and editing choices.

Investigating the different dynamics in Harris's *Nine Variations* and De Keersmaeker's and De Mey's *Rosa Danst Rosas* thus exemplifies how one might apply Laura Mulvey's theoretical propositions to the practice of screendance. Mulvey, for her own purposes, situated fetishism within a Freudian/Marxist matrix and with the central viewer identified as male/ heterosexual. If "cinema" is a mass art operating within a mainstream land-scape, dance and its meta-practices occupy the margins of mainstream culture.[19] Contemporary dance is largely a closed-system culture and one in which the demographics are decidedly unlike those of mainstream culture. Benedict Anderson, in his book *Imagined Communities*, reflects that com-munities, rather than being defined by geographical boundaries might also be considered contingent on common language. He proposes that a "sense of nationality" might survive beyond nation-states, preserved by language. If one extends this metaphor to the arts, and further to dance, then it is possible to propose that out of modern dance's leftist, socialist beginnings and its embrace of sexual indeterminacy, queer culture, and marginalized voices, the "gaze" of the viewer of screendance would be considerably at odds with Mulvey's "male gaze." In other words, in a practice so marginal-ized and so far from mainstream culture, it might be possible to assume that the male gaze would be neutralized.

Performance has been described by numerous theorists as having roots in ritual, in the transformative, and in the transcendent.[20] And where tech-nology became a fetish for artists, including the Dadaists, in the early years of the twentieth century, we now see a return to a similar fetishization in the digital age. As performance engages with the technological, it is often demystified, even secularized and is indeed reminiscent of the fascination with surfaces and technologically produced materials during Modernism as it eschewed metaphor and replaced it with brute formalism. The migration of live dance to the screen amplifies sexuality and nuance: the framing of intimate gestures amplifies tension. Regardless of the closed-system cul-ture in which contemporary screendance resides, the tendency toward fetishization of dancing bodies on screen persists. Bodies, whether coded as queer or straight, and certainly regardless of gender, are likely to be the object of *some* spectator's desire. It is the architecture of camera space itself that enables the presentation of any body as an object of desire, but that objectification is ultimately the collective purview of artists, curators, and consumers of screendance.

In her book *Screening the Body*, Lisa Cartwright notes that

> the motion picture, in conjunction with more familiar nineteenth-century medical recording and viewing instruments and techniques such as the kymograph, the microscope, and the X-ray apparatus, was a crucial instrument in the emergence of a distinctly modernist mode of representation in Western scientific and public culture—a mode geared to the temporal and spatial decomposition and reconfiguration of bodies as dynamic fields of action in need of regulation and control. It is a familiar claim in film scholarship that public audiences of the first motion pictures were thrilled by the body in motion. . . . Popular pleasure in the sight of moving bodies was bound up with the nineteenth-century development of recording instruments and graphic techniques that afforded scientists a degree of control over bodily movement not granted through, for example, the static technique of photography

The "popular pleasure" that Cartwright cites is all the more prevalent in the twenty-first century. Because video cameras are ubiquitous and digital culture makes all bodies equally accessible, either as images captured with cell phones or streaming pornography or videodance, there seems to be no limit to the pleasure we can extract from mediatized bodies. How then can we utilize this technology in the creation of art, and what, if anything, differentiates one digital body from another?

Cartwright continues, "cinematic apparatus can be considered as a cultural technology for the discipline and management of the human body."[21] This means that the technology of representation is also the technology of oppression. Given an informed appropriation of the power of technology to *mis*-represent, screendance does indeed offer the possibility for a kind of liberation from the laws of nature (such as gravity and temporality) via that very technology. If the body was "measured, regulated and reconceptualized in medicine and science" by the use of cinematic devices in the early part of the century, as Cartwright states, then I propose that screendance holds the potential to undo such cinematic oppression as a site for a kind of *liberated* body, one unhampered by the rigors of science or bound by the conventions of fetishization or objectification: instead, a screenic construction of a kinesthetic body freed from its sexualized, mediatized other. In the culture of contemporary dance, issues of gender, sexuality, and queer identity have been raised and deconstructed by numerous artists including Jane Comfort, Mark Dendy, Bill T. Jones and others. As it pertains to screendance, Mulvey's "male gaze" may evolve; but desire, voyeurism, and fetishism persist as the camera is a carnivore, consuming all it frames.

CHAPTER 10

Negotiating the Academy

Postmodernism has inexorably altered the rhetoric of higher education. Yet, while interdisciplinarity, a signature trait of postmodernism, is ostensibly highly valued in the academic environment, in most cases there is little actual overlap between the teaching of specific mediums or genres. In other words, mono-disciplinary areas of practice still persist and seem to be normative within universities and colleges. This adherence to disciplinary boundaries, while perhaps antithetical to the world of artistic practices outside of the academy, continues for many reasons. Some of those reasons are fiscal and budgetary; some are territorial and historical. Even so, screendance in the academy must seek out partners in order to emerge from the singular discipline of dance.

Finding such partners requires the navigation of territorial as well as geographical boundaries. Film, for instance—both practice and theory— might be taught in film or communication arts programs; video may be taught in communication arts or in the fine arts as an adjunct to time-based forms or "new genres"; and of course dance is taught within a dance department, sometimes associated with theater. Disciplinary compartmentalization requires considerable commitment on the part of the student, making it difficult for students to collaborate or to acquire skills outside of their specific area of study and often limiting the scope of their theoretical dialog. Screendance, as a hybrid and generally collaborative practice, thrives in an environment of interdisciplinarity and intertextuality, and as screendance tends to be diasporic in nature— that is, taking on the characteristics of its host site—the discipline from which academic courses emanate often pre-frames the language and critical analysis of the discourse surrounding the subject matter of screendance.

The provenance and scope of screendance courses available to students in a higher education environment varies greatly between institutions; in fact, there are very few university programs that confer degrees in screendance or associated areas of practice.[1] Due to both budgetary concerns and to the way in which universities introduce new degrees, screendance courses are often generated and taught by professors and teachers already within the university's teaching faculty, meaning that they have sometimes come to screendance through another artistic practice—quite often the practice of dance. This dynamic demonstrates the disciplinarily liminal state that screendance occupies: between being a new and foreign form of artistic expression, and being institutionally recognized. Such liminality is a product of the lag that occurs as academia decides whether to accept a particular new trend in the art world (or elsewhere) and whether to create curriculum that leads to a degree or focus in that nascent area of practice.

We can look, for example, to a similar moment in the late 1970s with the advent of video art and later with performance art. In 1971 David Ross was named the world's first curator of video art at the Everson Museum of Art in Syracuse, New York, well ahead of any degree granting programs in the subject. In fact, it was not until the end of the 1970s that video art was "integrated into academia through art, media art, and communication departments whose faculty members included early video practitioners" such as Suzanne Lacy, Jeanne C. Finley, Martha Rosler, and others.[2] This institutionalization of the form led to thriving video art communities across the United States and yielded festivals, museums, periodical literature, and galleries, all producing and disseminating the work of artists in a richly contextualized environment. It is clear that the intellectually stimulating gestalt that occurs when universities begin to support new and emerging forms of expression has ripple effects that resonate far beyond the walls of academia.

Again, though, the production of screendance and even its exhibition far outpaces its critical reception and academic institutionalization at this time. In order to consider the place of screendance in the academy, institutions must first clarify their rationale for its inclusion. They must ask whether the purpose of integrating screendance into existing curricula is designed to extend dance into another medium, thereby increasing the audience for dance, and whether moving-image technology is simply being marshaled as a support system for *re*-representing dance practice in a post-theater context. Or, is screendance being articulated within an academic setting as an interdisciplinary practice—of which dance is one discipline—along with other screen technologies, and also the appropriate theoretical and critical methodologies? If screendance is an iteration of dance training, it will most certainly be represented curricularly as such. If screendance is framed as an iteration of new media or video art practices, one can imagine that such an iteration would produce a different outcome.

This may seem obvious, but it is a distinction in need of attention. If, for instance, we think about screendance as an offshoot of film, then the lexicon and literature of film's history is a dominant curricular force. If we think about screendance as a subset of video art, then perhaps the literature and visual culture of that genre is the contextual foundation for a screendance course. In any case, the appropriate site for screendance in an academic setting is at the intersection of multiple disciplines, dance (of course) among them. Screendance is coming into academia at a time when interdisciplinarity is increasingly the lingua franca of many academic areas, and this makes it an ideal candidate to simultaneously fill multiple institutional needs, though inhabiting this role is also its greatest institutional challenge.

Because 35 or 16 mm film stock and its processing is prohibitively expensive, and as digital technologies have become the norm for media production, most moving-image courses found in universities—dance and art departments included—focus on *video* production. Additionally, since the late 1970s, a body of literature and criticism has evolved that supports video as an autonomous art form (video art), distinct from its numerous other uses and applications. As video production can be taught in the service of a widely diverse range of foci—including video art, narrative or experimental film, dance documentation, digital storytelling, or as support for the entertainment industry—it is important to clearly delineate the context within which a course will be situated. Video art, while generally historicized as a postwar art practice, is the product of an interdisciplinary history, so it would seem logical that as a subject in higher education it be located within an interdisciplinary or intermedia environment as well.[3] A video program with an interdisciplinary focus creates a fertile environment for students to not only acquire technological skills but also to put those skills into practice in work that crosses boundaries, genres, and mediums.[4]

Insofar as postmodern art practices routinely rely on collaboration, video is, in the contemporary art world, often the connective tissue that binds disparate disciplines together.[5] Video as tabula rasa is a pliant site that has historically occupied the center of an imaginary wheel from which virtually all of the postmodern art practices are connected, and out of which they radiate in some way or another. It has historically functioned as a site of documentation and also as a primary source of artistic expression for performative work; its malleability thus attracts all other time-based practices. It can be narrative or abstract, and it presents the possibility for endless reproduction and repeatability.

Since the advent of portable video technology in the mid 1960s, performance has been synergistically linked to its own recorded image. Indeed, much of the history of performance art is known only by grainy black-and-white videotapes. Artists who have been engaged with private, ritualistic performance actions, often undertaken with a small or nonexistent audience, have relied on mediated images of those actions as a kind of cultural capital, circulating as evidence of the original. As media has become ubiquitous, and technologies of representation and circulation have become increasingly accessible, the relationship of performance *to* media has further evolved into a number of site-specific practices. With this shift, the nature of performance itself is necessarily altered, through editing and the technologies by which performance is circulated within exhibition spaces and broadcast media.

Contemporary dance, for example, has identified media as a primary site of exploration, yielding screendance or dance made specifically for the camera. As dance migrates from its live performance to its mediated image, the private gesture—that which is created in the relative privacy of the camera's lens—is made public and amplified as it is broadcast or screened for an audience. The boundaries between media-contingent disciplines, however, are porous and fluid, and function more as place holders than restrictive prescriptions for any one approach or vision. Art made in the obscurity of classroom or university environments is a privilege of the academic environment, one that comes with teaching students in the relative shelter of academia. And while the teaching of video serves numerous functions in academia, the institutionalization of video and its relationship to performativity has a well-documented history.

Art historians, artists, and theorists of video have done an exceedingly good job of tracking that history, yet video has suffered from some of the same identity issues that screendance currently encounters. The video artist and scholar David Hall, writing about the early days of video in the UK, notes:

> difficulties arose when attempts were made to construct a rationale for an alternative, even "anti-modern," phase in video. While the popular new postmodernist debate addressed to other art activities remained within an understanding of the broad parameters of those activities, video art had by then

been all but lost in the confusion of a climate where arguments were made for its inclusion in a nebulous so-called video (or moving image) culture. Here problems occurred in attempting to critically identify new parameters for activities still evidently insisting on (though sometimes not admitting) a video art label, which, by their inclusion yet by definition, begged the question as to whether this was possible.[6]

Such paradoxes were and are a part of the evolution of any art form, particularly one that challenges existing cultural norms and is materially at odds with that which precedes it. This is a similar paradigm to that which universities must negotiate as they seek to include newer cultural manifestations within a curriculum.

But at what point should the academy seek to enter the discourse of an emerging art form such as screendance, and at what point should academia institutionalize a movement or genre, thereby risking the potential of ossifying it before it has been fully realized? Historicizing and institutionalizing any movement tends to curtail its forward motion. As a canon begins to take hold, and particular examples of work become the visual aids for university courses, the natural inclination toward mimesis begins to produce a multitude of copies. Perhaps this is inevitable; but in the earliest stages of a nascent academic subject, there is also the possibility that through a rigorous appraisal of the properties and desires of such a subject, one can articulate a literacy that includes both a visual culture and an evolving literature of the subject as well. One possibility for doing so is to begin to identify and describe trends in the field to this point, templates and subsets of the practice that have produced recognizable and quantifiable examples. Such examples may inform and enlarge the understanding of the practice of screendance. To properly frame screendance in an institutional setting requires an integrated course of study that situates the work in a broad context, one that may rely less on the histories of dance than other forms of art. In other words, if the inscription of dance (its own historicization) on film or video is the sole rationale for coursework in screendance, then screendance is relegated to being merely another way to extend dance into the popular culture. If the focus of academic screendance courses is on dance as an interdisciplinary, collaborative practice, articulating the site of activity within an entirely new paradigm, then by necessity the institutional literacy must engage in the kind of critical and theoretical analysis of screendance that film, video, and the visual arts have undergone in order to properly and fully chart this terrain.

What should a university course in screendance look like? It might look like a course in which dancing *or* non-dancing bodies are considered as part of an exploration of the moving image, an exploration and synthesis contextualized in equal parts by the history and practice of dance and the moving image, media theory, *and* dance theory, and art theories and histories as well. It would address the polemics of contemporary practices of technologically mediated bodies, and it would acknowledge that screendance is a by-product of the polyvocality of postmodern culture. It would not privilege postproduction over production or concept, and it would take into account that screendance is a part of the much larger canons and histories of video art and experimental film as well as contemporary dance. And it would be equal parts corporeal *and* technical—a screendance course would be a collaborative site where neither dance nor the method of mediation are given preference. In this way, boundaries might be broken and rigorous experimentation valued over and above a mimetic reproduction of existing models.

For university dance programs that endeavor to include media-based exploration of contemporary dance in their curriculum, fulfilling this prescription will necessitate a paradigm shift. And it is logical that a practice-specific curriculum, like dance, would foreground its own subject in all courses it offers. It is important to recognize that the history of screendance and its current practice is not necessarily initiated or produced through a dance gaze. It is not necessarily a picture of dance but a picture with dance *in it*. Universities are notorious for territorial battles, and while their rhetoric would lead us to believe that collaboration and interdisciplinarity are welcome, the entrenched paths to tenure and the way in which research and teaching are both assessed makes boundary-crossing difficult. Change comes slowly if at all, yet the value of activism during the process of screendance's institutionalization cannot be overstated.

Institutions of higher learning are historically slow to integrate avant-garde forms into their curriculum. Video and performance art are examples of two late twentieth-century additions to the "canon" that still struggle for acceptance in some academic institutions. The dance world beyond the walls of academia, though, is quite aware of the importance of, and the possibilities for video as an art form. As the most ephemeral of the art forms, dance is in a unique position to take advantage of video (and digital media in general), both as a tool for documentation and as a primary form of expression. As choreographers become more involved in media, and more literate in the specific language of the medium, screendance will become more and more viable as a genre of its own. Still, screendance has yet to be fully interrogated either within the university environment or in the context of contemporary art, and the literature framing screendance as a practice has not so far achieved a critical mass. Often, writing about screendance contextualizes the work as a subcategory of dance, or, in the case of Maya Deren and Shirley Clarke, as a tributary of experimental or independent film. Neither of these scenarios is completely satisfying, and both often fail to make new theory. The merging of dance and the optical mediums since the dawn of photography has traversed a wide and far-reaching territory, and along the way this merging has been shaped by the cultural manifestos of numerous movements, theorists, and philosophies. In practice, screendance has sought to liberate the dancing body from its own historical tethers and the often-oppressive weight of "dance" itself. To inscribe choreography within the finite, disjunctive medium of film or video is to break with dance and its reliance on the mythology of ephemerality. It is a radical act that is at odds with the nature of many theories and histories important to dance. The objectification of dance via media results in a kind of fixity and inscription, which forces a renegotiation of dance as a performance that relies upon liveness as its cultural capital. If dance is no longer considered as solely a "live art" form, then its relationship to media requires further negotiation. That negotiation must consider screendance and its subsets as well.

Screendance is contingent on, but is not, generically, dance. It is a practice outside of dance, a meta-practice. As such, screendance requires a kind of articulation beyond the frame of dance alone, one for which the critical vocabulary of dance is inadequate without additional support from disparate practices. This is not to say that a part of the discourse should *not* be dance theory, but that linking mediated images to only dance theory, history, and practice denies the oscillation between other equally or even more pertinent discourses. To articulate a theory of screendance, it is critical to engage dance theories with those residing outside the presumed scope of dance such as performance, visual art, film, and video as well as scholarship and histories of the moving image and mass culture, and modernist/postmodernist esthetics and cultural theories.[7] The inclusion of such theoretical discourse provides a foundation for looking at and talking about dance and its relationship to contemporary technology and its own mediated other. Contemporary art practice is not monolithic; instead, it is intertextual. Screendance would benefit from an embrace of historically relevant theory that opens the discourse to a more pluralistic interpretation of work in the field, while imposing a kind of analytic rigor often absent from the dialog. Much of the most important writing in the visual arts has historically come from artists themselves. The dance/technology/media community might benefit from the same sort of proactive, internal analysis of the state of the art. That is, if the theory does not exist, then perhaps the makers need to create it. This idea has been gaining traction in recent years as numerous artists in the field have begun engage in the production of both theoretical texts as well as practice-led research, symposia, conferences, and other community building around the idea of a more rigorous approach to screendance.[8]

Universities have generally become early adopters and consumers of new technologies, and although these technological "buy ins" are not necessarily done so in the support of new creative practices, they often inadvertently create spaces of opportunity for research and production of new art models. Thus, as dance has moved increasingly toward technology in its embrace of the digital domain, including digital and streaming video, interactive systems, multimedia applications, and the Internet, it has often done so while relying on the university's desire to be part of ongoing technological evolutions. The history of art and technology in the university environment begins in the early stages of the development of contemporary technologies of representation. In 1968, in the still-early days of video and performance art, the artist and professor Hans Breder established the graduate Intermedia Program at the University of Iowa.

> Soon the university became a key site for some of the period's most vital artists and writers, such as Allan Kaprow, Scott Burton, Willoughby Sharp, Hans Haacke, Robert Wilson, and Mary Beth Edelson. The opportunity to witness these artists and the experimental, participatory nature of the program were highly influential for a younger generation of artists.[9]

The program was also host to Elaine Summers, a participant in the earliest Judson Church activities who incorporated intermedia concepts into her work and subsequently established the Experimental Intermedia Foundation in New York. While in residence at Breder's program in 1973, Summers created two landmark dance film works, *Two Girls Downtown Iowa* and *Iowa Blizzard*.[10] This is an early model of the university as incubator for such work and one that is still relevant to media artists.

That trajectory was continued at the Institute for Studies in the Arts at Arizona State University in Tempe, which was a pioneer in interactive dance and the support of digitally mediated dance performance as well as the home of the Intelligent Stage. (see chapter 5) Although the Intelligent Stage and the Institute for Studies in the Arts were dismantled in 2003, they helped to initiate a new generation of experiments in dance and technology, training its participants not only in a technological skill set but in a theoretical one as well. It was an early model of artist-led research within the institutional setting of a university that has had historical resonance beyond its walls.

Creating dance and technology hybrids, including screendance, which are contingent on emerging technologies, allows makers to dematerialize the body in such a way as to cease its reliance on real time/space presence. It has becoming increasingly possible to create dance works in the digital realm that in fact require no "dancers" at all in the traditional sense. Using virtual space as the stage for these digital dances, choreographers and dance companies are questioning the very nature of dance in the postmodern/digital era. As such, they are part of a historical continuum of artists who engage technology, often in ways vastly different from its original or intended usage. Contemporary computing technologies have infiltrated universities and institutions in a way that makes possible any number of simultaneous users and/or organizational strategies that are well beyond the capabilities available only a few years ago. But incorporating technology into an academic course of study so as to differentiate it from software-driven or more generally mechanical uses of it requires a vigorous vision of its integration as an enabler of content.

Continuing to track the evolution of screendance in the university environment, much of the discourse surrounding screendance and dance, and technology in general, has taken place at a number of conferences and symposia. In 1992 the University of Wisconsin–Madison hosted the first International Dance and Technology Conference (IDAT). Since then, the conference has been held intermittently, most recently at York University in Toronto and at Arizona State University. The conference was an opportunity for artists working in the field to come together to present research in the form of papers, demonstrations, and performances. It was a fertile, often volatile environment where choreographers, technologists, and others, compared notes and discussed new developments in the field. Unfortunately, IDAT lost its momentum and no institution has sponsored it since 1999. In 2000, though, the University of Wisconsin–Madison held the first-ever conference on Dance for Camera, which has since been hosted by the American Dance Festival.[11] And there are many other conferences and symposia around the country, as well as in Europe, the U.K. and South America, that address pertinent issues related to screendance and new technologies in insightful and thoughtful ways. Much of the course material for university classes is gathered at these meetings, as professors and educators as well as practitioners can share their ideas, research, and responses to new developments in the field. More recent developments include The Centre for Screendance (http://arts.brighton.ac.uk/projects/screendance), hosted by the University of Brighton, and *The International Journal of Screendance* (http://journals.library.wisc.edu/index.php/screendance), published by Parallel Press at the University of Wisconsin-Madison.

Dance and technology and its numerous specific practices such as screen-dance have a kind of invisible history, one that is quite difficult to locate in the larger individual landscapes of either dance or art histories. That may be because screendance (for instance), being a collaborative process, is one in which the esthetics and histories of both the optical mediums and dance combine to create a new hybrid. In that hybrid, the individual histories of film, video, and dance are obscured and replaced by new and often uncharted histories. This is the history that must be mined in the university/institutional environment if screendance is to find a home in the academy.

Just as modernism's notion of the autonomy of the art object has been supplanted by indeterminacy and polyvocality, [12] so it may be that in the digital age, the merging of dance the moving image via digital technologies will lead to a new and more evolved understanding of dance and its mediated self. In order to do so, screendance must move on from its lengthy adolescence and begin to inscribe its particularities in academe in ways that are both cogent and articulate. To do so will thus blend the legacies of the historical and contemporary practice of screendance into the canons of both the visual arts and dance. Such gestures will insure that the literacy that flows from the screenic inscription of moving bodies is an accessible and challenging archive. It is in the interest of both dance and the media arts to continue to articulate that which screendance is as well as that which it is *not*, and that which separates it from documentation or theatrical work, or other dance and technology hybrids. In this way, we might continue to map and to trace the evolution of this distinct and vital hybrid form.

NOTES

PREFACE

1. Christine Elmo, "Christine Elmo on Artists Writing About Artists," *Critical Correspondence*. 5 January 2011. Web. http://www.movementresearch.org/criticalcorrespondence/blog/?p=2868. 13 May 2011.
2. Eisenstein was assigned a teaching position with the film school GIK (now Gerasimov Institute of Cinematography), and in 1933 and 1934 was in charge of writing curriculum. See "Sergei Eisenstein," on *Film Annex: Connect Through Film*. Web. 15 April 2011.
3. Mark Rothko, *The Artist's Reality: Philosophies of Art* (New Haven, CT: Yale University Press, 2004).
4. Judd's seminal essay, "Specific Objects," was a touchstone of theory for the formation of Minimalist aesthetics. In Stiles, Kristine and Peter Howard Selz. *Theories and Documents of Contemporary Art: A Sourcebook of Artists' Writings*. Berkeley: University of California Press, 1996. 114–117.
5. "Notes on Sculpture 1–3," originally published across three issues of *Artforum* in 1966; "Notes on Sculpture 4: Beyond Objects," originally published in *Artforum*, 1969.

INTRODUCTION

1. See Phillip Auslander, *Liveness: Performance in a Mediatized Culture* (New York: Routledge, 1999). More than simply archiving movement, media also codes and encodes movement.
2. See my article: "Video Space: A Site for Choreography," *LEONARDO: Journal of the International Society for the Arts, Sciences and Technology* 33.4 (2000): 275–80.
3. It is true that the terms "modernist" and "modernism" are now recognized as fluid and porous; nevertheless, both have entrenched and historically contingent meanings and are valuable semiotic markers for a particular approach to art making. I largely rely on Clement Greenberg's notion of modernism, as his has been the default definition for the latter part of the twentieth century to the present, and I use the term "modernist" to define difference in regard to materiality, especially in the context of the evolution toward postmodernism and its attendant philosophies.
4. There have been a number of positive developments in the field, including the recent Screendance Symposium, held at the University of Brighton in February 2011, which aimed to "present the conceptual framework of the recently launched International Journal of Screendance" and, through papers and presentations,

to "fuel the debates" surrounding the form. (See "Screendance Network" website, available at: http://artsresearch.brighton.ac.uk/research/projects/screendance-network/screendance-symposium-2011.

5. There are a few events that signal a movement toward increased critical discourse. In June 2006, Katrina McPherson, Simon Fildes, and Karl Jay-Lewin organized Opensource: {Videodance}, an artist-led, open symposium held in Findhorn, Scotland, for videodance makers and dance artists. The symposium, born out of a desire to "gather together a group [of videodance artists] to explore the issues upon which videodance's future depends [and to] develop a better dialogue between videodance artists to evolve a critical dialogue that is created and led by the makers and artists," featured four days of process-oriented discussion about the field and a number of guest speakers. See the Opensource conference website at <http://videodance.blogspot.com>. In July 2006 and 2008 I directed a four-day conference, Screendance: The State of the Art, at the American Dance Festival in Durham, North Carolina, intending to create a forum for rigorous discourse on the current state of screendance in the global community. The conference was attended by forty-five practitioners, scholars, educators, historians, and theorists from around the world, twenty-eight of whom presented papers on topics that theorized new ways of articulating the genre as well as historical narratives. In 2009 principal investigator Claudia Kappenberg, Brighton University was awarded an Arts and Humanities Research Counsel Grant to establish the International Screendance Network. One outcome of the two-year cycle of meetings and symposia was the founding of the first International Journal of Screendance. Web version available at: http://journals.library.wisc.edu/index.php/screendance

6. The art world seems increasingly interested in dance and its relationship to visual culture. I would note, for example, the appearance of the Trisha Brown Dance Company on the cover of *Artforum*'s January 2011 issue, as well as the inclusion of a number of choreographers in the recent (2010–11) exhibition On Line: Drawing Through the Twentieth Century at the Museum of Contemporary Art in New York.

7. There are certainly exceptions, though as seen in a number of festivals which have begun to include panels and seminars. However, these efforts are often driven by concerns outside of the theories put forth in this book.

8. While there is a serious lack of criticality in the United States, considerably more attention is paid to critical discourse in the UK, Canada, and Australia.

9. An exception to this point is the International Journal of Screendance as noted above.

10. Sidney Peterson, *The Avant-Garde Film: A Reader of Theory and Practice*, ed. P. Adams Sitney (New York: New York University Press, 1978), 75.

11. Ibid., 76, 75.

12. Jeffrey Bush and Peter Z. Grossman, "Videodance," *DanceScope* 9.2 (1975): 13.

13. Ibid., 12.

14. Ibid., 17.

15. Amy Greenfield, *Filmmakers Newsletter* 4.1 (Nov. 1970): 26.

16. Ibid., 27.

17. Ibid., 32.

18. Noël Carroll, "Toward a Definition of Moving-Picture Dance," in *Engaging the Moving Image* (New Haven, CT: Yale University Press, 2003), 236.

19. Two other excellent examples of a critique that works through intertextual lenses are Sally Banes's "Making Tharp Baryshnikov" and Sherril Dodds's *Dance on*

Screen: Genres and Media from Hollywood to Experimental Art. Banes applies a feminist analysis to Twyla Tharp's 1977 project, *Making Television Dance*; Dodds's
volume offers a number of analyses of video dance and dance for the camera works
filtered through contemporary theory. See Sally Banes, "Proceedings from the
'Dance for the Camera Symposium,'" (University of Wisconsin–Madison, 2000);
and Sherrill Dodds, *Dance on Screen: Genres and Media from Hollywood to
Experimental Art* (New York: Palgrave, 2001). There is increasingly more literature
on screendance being produced, including Judy Mitoma's *Envisioning Dance on
Film and Video* and Katrina McPherson's *Making Video Dance*. Yet while each of
these undoubtedly enhances the visibility of screendance, neither engages in the
kind of interdisciplinary critique that is necessary to the field's growth and viability. McPherson's volume is a practitioner's guide, which includes interviews with
leading contemporary video dance artists and is an invaluable resource for teaching the form of screendance. Mitoma's book, one of the first in the field, provides
an introduction to numerous screendance genres and an overview of dance for
screen, but it is largely dominated by noncritical essays by choreographers and
dancers who have worked in film and video. It thus repeats, in effect if not intention, the dance-centric perspective that remains persistent in the field.

20. The concept of "recorporealization" was first proposed in a paper presented at the
Dance for the Camera Symposium, held in Madison, Wisconsin, in February 2000,
wherein I defined recorporealization as "a literal *re*-construction of the dancing
body via screen techniques; at times a construction of an impossible body, one not
encumbered by gravity, temporal restraints or even death," (4). I subsequently
enlarged upon the concept in "Video Space: A Site for Choreography," *Leonardo*
33.4 (August 2000): 275–80.

1 ARCHIVES AND ARCHITECTURE

1. Ananda Mitra and Rae Lynn Schwartz, "From Cyber Space to Cybernetic Space:
Rethinking the Relationship between Real and Virtual Spaces," *Journal of
Computer-Mediated Communication* 7.1 (October 2001).
2. Sally Ann Ness, "The Inscription of Gesture: Inward Migrations in Dance," in
Migrations of Gesture, ed. Carrie Noland and Sally Ann Ness (Minneapolis:
University of Minnesota Press, 2008), 1–30, quotation on 1.
3. The boundaries between "film" as art and the art of advertising have been considerably blurred, and the delivery systems to which each belongs have considerable
overlaps as well.
4. Noël Carroll makes a very persuasive argument for another term "Motion Picture-
Dance" in *Engaging the Moving Image* (New Haven, CT: Yale University Press,
2003), 234–53. Carroll carefully crafts a case for his newly coined term that
artfully and analytically supports his assertion that motion picture–dance is the
most accurate term to describe the genre. However, the term does not roll off
the tongue well. So with the greatest respect to Carroll's study, I refer to the
practice as screendance in these pages.
5. Miwon Kwon, *One Place After Another: Site-Specific Art and Locational Identity*
(Cambridge, MA: MIT Press, 2004), 2.
6. Often footage shot in performance as documentation is modified in postproduction and juxtaposed or layered with other images made for the camera in an
attempt to utilize documentation footage more "artistically." Documentation footage is often created with poor camera position and lighting, and tends to "read" as
an afterthought in regard to screendance as a primary site of artistic production.

7. *El Fuego,* dir. Becky Edmunds, perf. A Gaucho. 2007; *Salt Drawing,* dir. Becky Edmunds, perf. Fiona Wright. 2004.

8. In the United States, programs such as PBS's *Great Performances* merge documentation with multiple camera editing in an attempt to find a middle ground between live performance and tele-visual dance broadcast. Another such endeavor, most frequently seen in Europe and Canada, is commissioned "dance for television," which is generally short-form film and video projects that are quickly cut and designed to keep the viewer engaged with the televised material.

9. Sherril Dodds, *Dance on Screen: Genres and Media from Hollywood to Experimental Art* (New York: Palgrave, 2001), 99.

10. Ibid., 9.

11. Walter Benjamin, "The Work of Art in the Age of Mechanical Reproduction," in *Modern Art and Modernism: A Critical Anthology*, ed. Francis Frascina and Charles Harrison (New York: The Open University, 1982), 217–27, quotation on 219.

12. Philip Auslander writes: "The . . . subsequent cultural dominance of mediatization has had the ironic result that live events now frequently are modeled on the very mediatized representations that once took the self-same live events as their models." *Liveness: Performance in a Mediatized Culture* (New York: Routledge, 1999), 10.

13. See Dodds, *Dance on Screen.*

14. Walter Benjamin was concerned that mechanical reproduction would diminish the value of the original. In his 1936 article he focused particular attention on the stage actor as he moved to acting for film:

> "The film actor," wrote Pirandello, "feels as if in exile—exiled not only from the stage but also from himself. With a vague sense of discomfort he feels inexplicable emptiness: his body loses its corporeality, it evaporates, it is deprived of reality, life, voice, and the noises caused by his moving about, in order to be changed into a mute image, flickering an instant on the screen, then vanishing into silence. The projector will play with his shadow before the public, and he himself must be content to play before the camera" (Luigi Pirandello, "Si Gira,", quoted by Leon Pierre-Quint, "Signification du cinema," in *L'Art cinematographique*, 14–15. This situation might also be characterized as follows: for the first time—and this is the effect of the film—man has to operate with his whole living person, yet forgoing its aura. For aura is tied to his presence; there can be no replica of it. The aura which, on the stage, emanates from Macbeth cannot be separated for the spectators from that of the actor. However, the singularity of the shot in the studio is that the camera is substituted for the public. Consequently, the aura that envelops the actor vanishes, and with it the aura of the figure he portrays. (219)

15. The New York Public Library for the Performing Arts and the Centre nationale de danse (CND) in France are two institutions with exhaustive video archives: they are essentially museums of the history of dance.

16. Amelia Jones, "'Presence' in Absentia: Experiencing Performance as Documentation," *Art Journal* 56.4 (1997): 11–18, quotation on 12.

17. Rosalind Krauss, "Video: The Esthetics of Narcissism," *October* 1 (1976): 50–64, quotation on 51.

18. Jacques Derrida, *Archive Fever: A Freudian Impression,* trans. Eric Prenowitz (Chicago: University of Chicago Press, 1995), 2.
19. Ibid., 2.
20. Ibid., 8.
21. Ibid., 18.
22. Ibid., 11.
23. See the definition of this term in my article "Video Space: A Site for Choreography," *Leonardo* 35.4 (2000).
24. Baudrillard writes: "The hyperreal represents a much more advanced stage insofar as it manages to efface even this contradiction between the real and the imaginary." *Jean Baudrillard, Selected Writings,* ed. Mark Poster (Stanford: Stanford University Press, 1988), 148.
25. Matthew Reason and Dee Reynolds, "Special Issue Editorial: Screen Dance Audiences—Why Now?" *Journal of Audience and Reception Studies* 7.2 (November 2010). Web. 24 February 2011.
26. While screendance may technically be constructed out of the ephemera of digital code (a cameraless construction), my main focus here is to articulate the architecture of the camera as both a particular method of mediation and a particular method of inscription.
27. See Charles M. Falco, "Use of optics by Renaissance artists." *McGraw Hill AccessScience: Encyclopedia of Science & Technology Online.* Web. 20 March 2010.
28. Harry Shunk, "Leap into the Void." Photograph, 1960, Metropolitan Museum of Art, New York. (Harry Shunk and John Kender montaged a series of photographs, including with and without the cyclist in the background, and one of Klein diving off the wall and onto a pile of cushions.)
29. David Vaughan, "Locale: The Collaboration of Merce Cunningham and Charles Atlas." *Millennium Film Journal* 10/11 (1981–82): 18–22, quotation on 20.
30. Ibid., 6.
31. Marshall McLuhan, "The Medium Is the Message," in *Essential McLuhan,* ed. Eric McLuhan and Frank Zingrone (New York: Basic Books, 1995), 151.

2 MEDIATED BODIES

1. See Noël Carroll, *Toward a Definition of Moving-Picture Dance: Engaging the Moving Image.* New Haven, CT: Yale University Press, 2003.
2. Judy Mitoma, ed., *Envisioning Dance on Film and Video,* (New York: Routledge, 2002).
3. Sherril Dodds, *Dance on Screen: Genres and Media from Hollywood to Experimental Art* (New York: Palgrave, 2001), 1–29.
4. Noël Carroll argues for the establishment for "objective classifications of artworks." He writes: "when we fix the category to which an artwork belongs, we avail ourselves of the means for assessing whether or not the work is good of its kind." Carroll, *On Criticism* (New York: Routledge, 2009), 9. In order for works of art—in this case, screendance—to be included in timelines or given "landmark" status, and to avoid overreliance on "taste," there needs to be a logical application of critical standards.
5. The Institute of Contemporary Art in Philadelphia held an exhibition called Dance With Camera from September 11, 2009 to March 21, 2010. The press release read, "With iconic dance films, ranging from Busby Berkeley's Hollywood musicals to Maya Deren's avant-garde films, the screenings in this cinema program exemplify

the ways dance has compelled visual artists to record bodies moving in time and space." Even though the curator chose other works to screen as well, Berkeley and Deren became, by default, the representative poles of the practice. In Sherril Dodds's *Dance on Screen: Genres and Media from Hollywood to Experimental Art*, the author describes Hollywood's domination of the film industry in the 1930s via its creation of the "musical" (5); she then states: "One of the most interesting aspects of the musical genre is that dance routines were choreographed specifically for the film medium, and Busby Berkeley was one director who filmed dance in an innovative way." Two pages later, turning her attention to the "avant-garde," Dodds says: "One of the most significant film-makers, located within the avant-garde, in relation to dance on film is Maya Deren, [who is] cited as being the innovator of 'choreo-cinema' an art form in which dance and the camera are inextricably linked" (7). Dodds, *Dance On Screen: Genres and Media from Hollywood to Experimental Art* (New York: Palgrave, 2001).

6. The architectural specificity of the camera is a much more complex space than "media," and it is also a site-specific space. "Media" is not a site but rather a catch-all phrase used to describe any number of communication technologies. Furthermore, the designations commonly used interchangeably, such as video-dance, dance film, and the like are materially specific; that is, they locate dance in a specific technology such as video or film and as such those technologies have historical weight as well as specific characteristics and properties.

7. For a further discussion of the relationship between the phenomenology of train travel and dance, see Felicia M. McCarren's chapter "The Dancer, the Train, and the Cinema," in *Dancing Machines: Choreographies in the Age of Mechanical Reproduction* (Stanford, CA: Stanford University Press, 2003), 43–44.

8. For more on Muybridge, see Kevin MacDonnell, *Eadweard Muybridge: The Man Who Invented the Moving Picture* (London: Weidenfield and Nicolson, 1972); *Gordon Hendricks: Eadweard Muybridge: The Father of the Motion Picture* (London: Secker and Warburg, 1975); Rebecca Solnit, *River of Shadows: Eadweard Muybridge and the Technological Wild West* (New York: Viking, 2003); Brian Clegg, *The Man Who Stopped Time: The Illuminating Story of Eadweard Muybridge: Pioneer Photographer, Father of the Motion Picture, Murderer* (Washington, D.C., Joseph Henry Press, 2007).

9. Matthew Josephson, *Edison: A Biography* (New York: McGraw-Hill, 1959), 386.

10. For more on Edison's film work, see Ronald W. Clark, *Edison: The Man Who Made the Future* (New York: G. P. Putnam's Sons, 1977); Neil Baldwin, *Edison: Inventing the Century* (New York: Hyperion, 1995); Charles Musser, "At the Beginning: Motion Picture Production, Representation and Ideology at the Edison and Lumière Companies," in *The Silent Cinema Reader*, ed. Lee Grieveson and Peter Krämer (New York: Routledge, 2004).

11. While Muybridge is often missing from conversations regarding screendance, he has been the subject of considerable attention in the dance and multimedia/art communities. See review of Philip Glass's multimedia piece about Muybridge's life, "The Photographer: Far from Truth" in the *New York Times* (John Rockwell, "Philip Glass's 'Photographer.'" *New York Times*, 7 October 1983. Web. http://www.nytimes.com/1983/10/07/arts/philip-glass-s-photographer.html?scp=1&s. 15 April 2011.)

12. Roland Barthes, *Camera Lucida: Reflections on Photography*, trans. Richard Howard (New York: Hill and Wang, 1981), 15.

13. See Virginia Brook's chapter, "From Méliès to Streaming Video: A Century of Moving Dance Images," in Mitoma, *Envisioning Dance*, 54–60. Also see Erin Brannigan,

"Modern Movement, Dance, and the Birth of Cinema," in *Dancefilm: Choreography and the Moving Image* (Oxford: Oxford University Press, 2011), 19–38.

14. For more on Méliès, see Elizabeth Ezra, *George Méliès: The Birth of the Auteur* (New York: Manchester University Press, 2000).

15. Amy Greenfield, "The Kinesthetics of Avant-Garde Dance Film: Deren and Harris," in Mitoma, *Envisioning Dance*, 23.

16. Tom Gunning, "Chaplin and the Body of Modernity," (conference proceedings, *The BFI Charles Chaplin Conference*, July 2005). Web. 13 March 2011.

17. As I have noted, Charlie Chaplin aptly demonstrated the capacity for film and dance to elevate each other into a hybrid, performative space (though in Chaplin's case, dance as an idiosyncratic, personal and even quotidian movement vocabulary). In Chaplin's films, movement created for the camera interrupted narrative flow and reinforced cinema's ability to place multiple modes of artistic practice inside of a single frame.

18. Roger Copeland, "Merce Cunningham and the Politics of Perception," in *What is Dance? Readings in Theory and Criticism*, ed. Roger Copeland and Marshall Cohen (London: Oxford University Press, 1983), 313.

19. Copeland, *The Modernizing of Modern Dance* (New York: Routledge, 2004), 110.

20. Frederick Jameson, *Postmodernism, or, The Cultural Logic of Late Capitalism* (Durham, NC: Duke University Press 1991), 74.

21. Maya Deren, *An Anagram of Ideas on Art, Form and Film* (Yonkers, NY: The Alicat Book Shop Press, 1946), 6, 5.

22. Erin Brannigan, "Yvonne Rainer," *Senses of Cinema* 27 (July–August 2003). Web. 18 November 2007.

23. Sally Banes, *Dancing Women: Female Bodies on Stage* (New York: Routledge, 1998), 222.

24. Brannigan, "Yvonne Rainer," Web. 24 February 2011.

3 RECORPOREALIZATION AND THE MEDIATED BODY

1. Hal Foster, *The Return of the Real: The Avant-Garde at the End of the Century* (Cambridge, MA: MIT Press, 1996).

2. Rebecca Solnit, *River of Shadows: Eadweard Muybridge and the Technological Wild West* (New York: Penguin Books, 2003), 4, 115.

3. Akira Mizuta Lippit, *Migrations of Gesture* (Minneapolis: University of Minnesota Press, 2008), 116.

4. Ibid., 117.

5. Michael Rush, *New Media in Late 20th-Century Art* (London: Thames and Hudson, 1999), 13–14.

6. Margot Lovejoy, *Postmodern Currents: Art and Artists in the Age of Electronic Media*. 2nd ed. (Upper Saddle River, NJ: Prentice Hall, 1997), 29.

7. Rush, *New Media*, 19.

8. Allan Kaprow, *Essays on the Blurring of Art and Life*, ed. Jeff Kelley, rev. ed. (Los Angeles: University of California Press, 2003), 7–9.

9. Sally Banes, *Terpsichore in Sneakers* (Hanover, NH: University Press of New England, 1977/1987), 10.

10. Lucy Lippard, *Six Years: The Dematerialization of the Art Object from 1966 to 1972* (Los Angeles: University of California Press, 1997), xi.

11. See Banes, "Introduction: Sources of Post-Modern Dance," in *Terpsichore in Sneakers*.

12. As Susan Sontag writes in *On Photography*: "It could be argued . . . that the very situation which is not determinative of taste in photography, its exhibition in

museums and galleries, has revealed that photographs do possess a kind of authenticity." (New York: Anchor Books/Doubleday, 1989), 139–40.

13. See Kaprow *Essays on the Blurring of Art and Life*.
14. Ibid., 195.
15. Ibid., 195.
16. Lovejoy, *Postmodern Currents*, 39.
17. John Berger, *About Looking* (New York: Pantheon Books, 1980), 50.
18. See: <http://seul-le-cinema.blogspot.com/2009/08/films-i-love-40-9-variations-on-dance.html>
19. Roland Barthes, *Roland Barthes*, trans. Richard Howard (London: Macmillan, 1977), 36.
20. Sally Ann Ness, *Migrations of Gesture* (Minneapolis: University of Minnesota Press, 2008), 1.
21. Walter Benjamin, *Reflections: Essays, Aphorisms, Autobiographical Writings,* ed. Peter Demetz (New York: Schocken Books, Inc.), 229.
22. To the other extreme, in work that is not a product of real bodies performing for the camera (i.e., movement that is derived from completely digital or synthetic data and so corporealized for the first time),we encounter the digital simulacra of dancing bodies that recall for us the very real difference between the expressivity of human beings moving in space and their mnemonic mediatized artifacts. The same observation might be made in regard to work derived from motion capture and other such contemporary technologies of representation.
23. John Joseph Martin, *John Martin's Book of the Dance* (New York: Tudor, 1963), 138.
24. Ibid.
25. See Sontag, *On Photography*.
26. Roland Barthes, *Camera Lucida: Reflections on Photography* (New York: Hill and Wang, 1980), 81.
27. Walter Benjamin, "The Work of Art in the Age of Mechanical Reproduction," in *Modern Art and Modernism: A Critical Anthology*, ed. Francis Frascina and Charles Harrison (New York: The Open University, 1982), 233.
28. *Untitled,* chor./perf. Bill T. Jones; text: Arnie Zane, Bill T. Jones; dir. John Sanborn, Mary Perillo; prod. Debbie Lepsinger; music by Hector Berlioz. Produced for "Live From Off Center," KTCA-TV, Minneapolis, MN, 1989.
29. Richard Schechner, *Performance Theory*, rev. ed. (New York: Routledge, 1988), 120.

4 THE ADVENT OF VIDEO CULTURE

1. See Philip Auslander, *Liveness: Performance in a Mediatized Culture* (New York: Routledge, 1999).
2. Lindsy E. Pack, *The Ernie Kovacs Show* (various episodes): U.S. Comedy/Variety Program." *The Museum of Broadcast Communications*. Web.
3. "Tele-visual" is a term borrowed from Sherril Dodds's *Dance on Screen*, in which she refers to the "tele-visual apparatus in the construction of motion within screen dance." (New York: Palgrave, 2001), 28.
4. Michael Arlen, *Living-Room War* (Syracuse, NY: Syracuse University Press, 1997), 8.
5. Ibid.
6. Numerous artists, including Michael Heizer and Robert Smithson, have sited works of art in the landscape as opposed to within the museum or gallery

system, thus necessitating that viewers travel to the space upon which the work is contingent.

7. The "first person" refers to an acknowledgement of the camera's gaze by the performer (in other words the performer literally makes "eye contact" with the camera), thus breaking Brecht's "fourth wall." The "third person" refers to a scenario in which the camera is a passive witness to all that flows across its field of vision, and/or the gaze is voyeuristic.

8. See chap. 6 for a discussion of Rainer's *NO Manifesto*.

9. Rose Lee Goldberg, *Performance: Live Art: 1909 to the Present* (Ann Arbor: University of Michigan Press, 1979), 94.

10. Ibid.

11. Henry M. Sayre, *The Object of Performance: The American Avant-Garde since 1970* (Chicago: University of Chicago Press, 1989), 204.

12. See Miwon Kwon, *One Place After Another: Site-Specific Art and Locational Identity* (Boston: MIT Press, 2004).

13. *Quarry*, dir. Meredith Monk. Black and White. Silent, 5.3 Minutes, 16 mm. The film was designed to be projected in the performing space during presentation of Monk's opera *Quarry*, but has been screened apart from the opera as well.

14. See Sayre, *Object of Performance*.

15. Erin Brannigan, *Dancefilm: Choreography and the Moving Image* (Oxford: Oxford University Press, 2011), 94.

16. During her life Bausch worked in media in a number of capacities. *The Lament of the Empress* (also translated as *The Plaint of the Empress)*, was directed by Bausch and filmed on location in Wuppertal, Germany, between October 1987 and April 1989 (originally shot on 35 mm film).Bausch was the subject of a number of documentaries, including one by the director Chantal Akerman, *Un jour Pina a Demandé* (*One Day Pina Asked*) from 1983, and more recently *Dancing Dreams*, directed by Anne Linsel and Rainer Hoffmann, and Wim Wenders's 3D film, *Pina*, completed subsequent to the choreographer's death.

17. Brannigan, *Dancefilm*, 94.

18. While I recognize the provenance of gesture and narrative drama as developed by D. W. Griffith, and other early filmmakers, the techniques Griffith drew from were most certainly based in mimicry and the theatrical techniques of the era. What is often generalized as "filmic" or "cinematic" in contemporary dance and or screendance has less to do with Griffith—or Eisenstein, for that matter—than with the art of the actual era during which individual works for theater or screen are created.

19. Bernhard Giesen, "Performance Art," in *Social Performance: Symbolic Action, Cultural Pragmatics, and Ritual*, ed. Jeffrey C. Alexander, Bernhard Giesen, and Jason L. Mast (Cambridge University Press, 2006), 315–24.

20. Ibid., 316

21. For example, work shot in film is often referred to as "video dance" while "cine-dance" or "dance film" would be more accurate.

22. Woody Vasulka quoted in Jon Burris, "Did the Portapak Cause Video Art? Notes On the Formation of a New Medium," *Millennium Film Journal* 29 (Fall 1996): 3–28, quotation on 4.

23. Burris, "Did the Portapak Cause Video Art?.

24. See Douglas Rosenberg, "Video Space: A Site for Choreography," *Leonardo* 33.4 (2000): 275–80.

25. Edith Decker-Phillips, *Paik Video* (Barrytown, NY: Barrytown LTD, 1998), 60.

26. See Mary Ann Kearns, "The Role of Technology in the Art of Nam June Paik: Paik's Videotapes," *The Experimental Television Center's Video History Project*. Web. 1988.

27. Quoted in Toni Stoos and Thomas Kellein, eds., *Nam June Paik: Video Time, Video Space* (New York: H. N. Abrams, 1998), 36.

28. Doug Hall and Sally Jo Feiffer, *Illuminating Video: An Essential Guide to Video Art* (Ann Arbor: University of Michigan Press, 1990), 14.

29. Anna Kisselgoff, "Dance: Joanne Kelley (sic) With Tape," *New York Times*, November 20, 1977, 67.

30. Kathy High writes: "Twenty-five years ago, a seminal program called the Television Laboratory (TV Lab) was sponsored by Thirteen/WNET (co-sponsored by KQED in San Francisco and WGBH in Boston, and funded by the Rockefeller Foundation, NYSCA, and the NEA). Under the directorship of David Loxton (and later under the co-directorship of Carol Brandenberg), TV Lab functioned as a workshop. Thirteen/WNET opened up its broadcast studio facilities to video artists, who could experiment with their equipment throughout the year. Works produced at the TV Lab were used either purely for research or for broadcast. Out of TV Lab came productions that were radically off-center from other television programming, and that today are landmarks in the history of independent video and the medium of television." "On REEL NEW YORK," *Thirteen: WNET New York*. Web. 3 March 2011.

31. For example, Donald McKayle's "Rainbow 'Round my Shoulder" was broadcast on CBS Camera 3 Live Television in 1959.

32. See Noël Carroll, *A Philosophy of Mass Art* (New York: Oxford University Press, 1998).

33. See Donald F. Theall and Edmund Carpenter, *The Virtual Marshall McLuhan* (Montreal: McGill-Queen's University Press, 2001), 167–68.

34. Mark Federman, "What is the Meaning of the Medium is the Message?" Web. 4 January 2010.

35. Ibid.

5 THE BRIDE IS DANCE

1. Calvin Tomkins, *Duchamp: A Biography* (New York: Henry Holt and Company, Inc., 1996), 297.

2. While I acknowledge that this gendered construction is problematic, I use it as a metaphor found in Duchamp's work in order to make a point about the way in which technology consumes performance. In the culture of contemporary dance, issues of gender, sexuality, and queer identity have been raised and deconstructed by numerous artists including Jane Comfort, Mark Dendy, Bill T. Jones, and others, rendering "male gaze" to a large degree as the *spectator's* gaze. Further and more broadly, mediated dance, aggressively recontextualized as it is by technology, actually exacerbates the conditions for desire, voyeurism, and fetishism.

3. For another similar example, we look to Hinton's later collaboration with Rosemary Lee, called *Snow* (2003), in which archival footage of people performing winter activities such as ice-skating is edited together to create a screen choreography.

4. "At the premiere some listeners were unaware that they had heard anything at all. It was first performed . . . for an audience supporting the Benefit Artists Welfare Fund—an audience that supported contemporary art. . . . Cage said, 'People began whispering to one another, and some people began to walk out. They didn't laugh—they were just irritated when they realized nothing was going to happen,

and they haven't forgotten [*sic*] it 30 years later: they're still angry.' . . . To Cage, silence had to be redefined if the concept was to remain viable. He recognized that there was no objective dichotomy between sound and silence, but only between the intent of hearing and that of diverting one's attention to sounds. "'The essential meaning of silence is the giving up of intention,'" he said. This idea marks the most important turning point in his compositional philosophy. He redefined silence as simply the absence of intended sounds, or the turning off of our awareness." Larry J. Solomon, "The Sounds of Silence: John Cage and 4'33," *Media Art Net*, 15 October 2010. Web. 2002.

5. Perhaps as a result the ubiquitous presence of moving images in contemporary life, the presence of media within a theatrical environment now encounters little resistance. Dance audiences are accustomed to experiencing dance and music simultaneously; however, it is a more recent experience for many to encounter dance and *moving image* media simultaneously sharing the same space. Although artists have long experimented with "filmic" space in live performance—going back to the work of Elaine Summers and others in the 1960s—the practice did not reach a critical mass until recently, with the availability of easily accessible video projectors, laptops, and user-friendly output hardware and software. There also seems to be little resistance anymore (by audiences) to the split stream of focus and multiple narratives or streams of consciousness that accompany many contemporary dance/media hybrids performances.

6. Hal Foster, *The Return of the Real: The Avant-Garde at the End of the Century* (Cambridge: MIT Press, 1996).

7. "Telematics is a term used to designate computer-mediated communications networking involving telephone, cable, and satellite links between geographically dispersed individuals and institutions that are interfaced to data-processing systems, remote sensing devices, and capacious data storage banks." Roy Ascott, "Is There Love in the Telematic Embrace?" *Art Journal* 49, no 3: (Fall 1990): 241.

8. Amelia Jones, "Presence in Absentia: Experiencing Performance as Documentation-Performance Art Focusing on the Human Body in the Early 1960s Through the 1970s," *Art Journal* 56, no. 4 (Winter 1997): 11–18, quotation on 12.

9. Ibid., 14.

10. Ascott, "Is There Love?" 241–47, quotation on 243.

11. Lev Manovich, *The Language of New Media* (Boston: MIT Press, 2002), 61.

12. Susan Sontag, *Against Interpretation and Other Essays* (New York: Picador, 1966), 3.

13. Ibid., 4, 5.

14. Ibid., 5.

15. Ibid., 6.

16. Ibid., 6.

17. Ibid., 7.

18. Ascott, "Is There Love?" 241.

6 EXCAVATING GENRES

1. See Benedict Anderson's *Imagined Communities* (New York: Verso, 1983).

2. Noël Carroll, *On Criticism* (New York: Routledge, 2009). 72.

3. Such attempts have been made, as early as 2000, via conferences that focus on screendance.

4. Sherril Dodds, *Dance on Screen: Genres and Media from Hollywood to Experimental Art* (New York: Palgrave, 2001), 25.

5. Marcel Duchamp writes: "All in all, the creative act is not performed by the artist alone; the spectator brings the work in contact with the external world by deciphering and interpreting its inner qualifications and thus adds his contribution to the creative act," quotation in Gyorgy Kepes, *The Visual Arts Today* (Middletown, CT: Wesleyan University Press, 1960), 111–12.
6. Claudia Kappenberg, "Does Screendance Need to Look Like Dance?" *International Journal of Performance Arts and Digital Media* (hereafter *PADM*) 5, nos. 2–3 (2009): 89–105, quotation on 91.
7. The festival that I direct at the American Dance Festival was called "Dancing For the Camera: International Festival of Film and Video Dance." It was so-named more than fifteen years ago, but in 2011 the name was changed to the International Festival of Screendance to reflect a different understanding of the form.
8. *Dance on Camera*, a slight variation, has similar resonance, though the probable meaning here is a combination of dance *for camera* and *dance on screen*. Claudia Kappenberg notes that "The home page for the annual 'Dance on Camera Festival' in New York demonstrates this legacy, stating that since its creation in 1971, its mission has been to facilitate the preservation of dance, encourage documentaries on dance and further screen adaptations. I would argue that all three categories are representative of a 'dance for film' approach in that the film-making and its technologies are predominantly put at the service of the dance." Kappenberg, "Does Screendance Need to Look Like Dance?" 93.
9. Michael Kirby and Sally Banes, Introduction. *Drama Review* 19 (March 1975): 3.
10. Sally Banes, *Terpsichore in Sneakers,* Hanover, NH: University Press of New England, 1977/1987), xiii.
11. See for example Rose Lee Goldberg's *Performance Art: From Futurism to the Present,* rev. ed. (New York: Harry N. Abrams, 1988), 3.
12. The "Vows of Chastity" read:
    1. Filming must be done on location. Props and sets must not be brought in. If a particular prop is necessary for the story, a location must be chosen where this prop is to be found.
    2. The sound must never be produced apart from the images or vice versa. Music must not be used unless it occurs within the scene being filmed, i.e., diagetic.
    3. The camera must be a hand-held camera. Any movement or immobility attainable in the hand is permitted. The film must not take place where the camera is standing; filming must take place where the action takes place.
    4. The film must be in colour. Special lighting is not acceptable (if there is too little light for exposure the scene must be cut or a single lamp be attached to the camera).
    5. Optical work and filters are forbidden.
    6. The film must not contain superficial action (murders, weapons, etc. must not occur.)
    7. Temporal and geographical alienation are forbidden (that is to say that the film takes place here and now).
    8. Genre movies are not acceptable.
    9. The final picture must be transferred to the Academy 35mm film, with an aspect ratio of 4:3, that is, not widescreen. Originally, the requirement was that the film had to be *filmed* on Academy 35mm film, but the rule was relaxed to allow low-budget productions.
    10. The director must not be credited.

Mette Hjort and Scott MacKenzie, eds., *Purity and Provocation: Dogma 95* (London: British Film Institute, 2003), 199–200.

13. Katrina McPherson, Litza Bixler, and Deveril. *left-luggage.co.uk.* "Dogma Dance." 18 August 2007. Web. 12 March 2010.

14. Deveril, message posted on "Dance and Technology" listserv. Web. Accessed 12 March 2010.

15. Ibid.

16. See Douglas Rosenberg's 1999 manifesto in Hjort and MacKenzie, *Purity and Provocation: Dogma 95*, 173.

17. Henry M. Sayre, *Object of Performance: The American Avant-garde Since 1970* (Chicago: University of Chicago Press, 1989), xii.

18. Bill Nichols, ed., *Maya Deren and the American Avant-Garde* . (Berkeley: University of California Press, 2001), 131–50.

19. Ibid., 141.

20. Ibid.

21. This use of the work "screenic" was introduced to the screendance network in discussion by Harmony Bench. It has also appeared in common usage in place such as N. Katherine Hayles, "Print Is Flat, Code Is Deep: The Importance of Media-Specific Analysis," *Poetics Today* 25, no. 1 (Spring 2004): 67–90. Hayles writes: "In the computer, the signifier exists not as a durably inscribed flat mark but as a screenic image produced by layers of code precisely correlated through correspondence rules, from the electronic polarities that correlate with the bit stream to the bits that correlate with binary numbers, to the numbers that correlate with higher-level statements, such as commands, and so on. Even when electronic hypertexts simulate the appearance of durably inscribed marks, they are transitory images that need to be constantly refreshed by the scanning electron beam that forms an image on the screen to give the illusion of stable endurance through time" (74).

22. *Diagonale Symphonie* is viewable online at: http://www.ubu.com/film/eggeling.html.

23. Statement at beginning of film by Frederick J. Kiesler, a noted designer and writer associated with the Surrealists.

24. See Richard Suchenski, "Hans Richter," in *Senses of Cinema*. Web. 15 March 2010. http://www.sensesofcinema.com/2009/great-directors/hans-richter/.

25. See for instance, Mary Ann Caws, ed., *Manifesto: A Century of Isms* Lincoln: University of Nebraska Press, 2000).

26. See Douglas Rosenberg, "Curating the Practice/The Practice of Curating." *PADM* 5, nos. 2–3 (December 2009): 75–87.

27. Susan Hayward, *Cinema Studies: The Key Concepts*, 2nd. ed. (New York: Routledge, 2000), quotation on 151.

28. Erin Brannigan, "Micro-choreographies: The Close-up in Dancefilm," *PADM* 5, nos. 2–3 (December 2009): 121–39, quotation on 126.

29. Ibid., 126–27.

30. Kappenberg, "Does Screendance Need to Look Like Dance?" 90.

7 CURATING THE PRACTICE/THE PRACTICE OF CURATING

1. Andre Lepecki, *Exhausting Dance: Performance and the Politics of Movement* (New York: Routledge, 2006), 5.

2. Ibid., 5.

3. Geoff Cox and Joasia Krysa. "O zadaniach kuratorw wobec obiektw niemateri-alnych: generowanie I uszkadzanie obiektw cyfrowych" ("Immaterial Curating: the

generation and corruption of the digital object"), trans. Marta Walkowiak. In Lukasz Ronduda, ed., *Zeszyty Artystyczne* 11 (Poznan: Uniwersytet Poznanski), 104–15.

4. There are certainly exceptions to this observation in the screendance community including the *What If... festival* (www.whatiffestival.co.uk), (2010) A festival drawing from work in film, dance, live and visual art co-curated by five artists with a background in dance, visual art and film-making: Lucy Cash, Becky Edmunds, Claudia Kappenberg and Chirstinn Whyte. My own engagement with curating screendance goes back to an exhibition of more than one hundred works for screen as part of the 1999 *International Dance and Technology Conference,* Arizona State University, Tempe, Arizona. Other notable exceptions are James Byrne's curated screenings at Dance Theater Workshop in New York, *Eyes Wide Open* (1989), and Amy Greenfield/Elaine Summers seminal *FILMDANCE* (1983). At present, two other endeavors also come to mind. The first is an ongoing salon style event in Williamsburg, New York, presented by Kinetic Cinema and curator Anna Brady Nuse and others; the second, a museum exhibition curated by Jenelle Porter at the University of Pennsylvania's Institute of Contemporary Art, which was on exhibit September 11, 2009–March 21, 2010. The ICA exhibition was an example of the tendency to rely on such institutionalized narratives that place Maya Deren, *Singin' in the Rain*, and Busby Berkeley in the same context as Yvonne Rainer and Norman McLaren. Finally, I would also note the work of Paulo Caldas, Eduardo Bonito, and Regina Levy, producers of the *Dança em foco* festival in Brazil, as well as the efforts of Portland Green Cultural Projects (http://www.portland-green.com). Also of note is Nuria Font in Barcelona who has been a great advocate for the field.Katrina McPherson and Simon Fildes in Scotland and Ellen Bromberg in Utah continue to advocate for curation as a model for new knowledges in the field.

5. See for example www.on-curating.org, an online journal devoted to discussions of curating and its relative importance to the visual arts.

6. Liz Wells, "Curatorial Strategy as Critical Intervention: The Genesis of Facing East," in *Issues in Curating Contemporary Art and Performance,* ed. Judith Rugg and Michele Sedgwick (Chicago: University of Chicago Press, 2008), 29–45, quotation on 29.

7. Lois H. Silverman, "Making Meaning Together: Lessons from the field of American History," in *Reinventing the Museum: Historical and Contemporary Perspectives on the Paradigm Shift*, ed. Gail Anderson (Oxford: Rowman and Littlefield Publishers, Inc., 2004), 233–42.

8. Paul. O'Neill, "The Curatorial Turn: From Practice to Discourse," in Rugg and Sedgwick, *Issues in Curating,* 14–15.

9. Clement Greenberg, "Avant-Garde and Kitsch," in *The Collected Essays and Criticism: Perceptions and Judgments, 1939–1944, Volume 1,* ed. John O'Brian (Chicago: University of Chicago Press, 1986), 5–22, quotation on 6.

10. See Theodor Adorno, *The Culture Industry*. New York: Routledge, 2001.

11. Greenberg, "Avant-Garde and Kitsch," 11.

12. The following is a partial list of international screendance festivals: Dance for the Camera (Chicago); Dance on Camera Festival (New York); Videodansa, Barcelona Prize (IDN) (Spain); Festival of Dance and Electronic Media (Mexico), DANCEonFILM (San Diego/Tijuana); Dance Camera West (Los Angeles); ScreenDance Park Gallery Falkirk (Scotland); International Dance Video Festival (Yokohama), Constellation Change Screen Dance Festival (UK); Dance Camera (Istanbul).

13. Yvonne Rainer, "Some Retrospective Notes on a Dance for 10 People and 12 Mattresses Called Parts of Some Sextets," in *Happenings and Other Acts*, ed. Mariellen R. Sandford (London: Routledge, 1995), 130–37.

14. Sally Banes, *Terpsichore in Sneakers* (Hanover, NH: University Press of New England, 1977/1987), 43.

15. Jeff Kelley, *Childsplay: The Art of Allan Kaprow* (Berkeley: University of California Press, 2004), 51.

16. See Sally Banes, *Writing Dancing in the Age of Postmodernism* (Middletown, CT: Wesleyan University Press, 1994), 208–19.

17. See for example Philip Auslander, *Liveness: Performance in a Mediatized Culture.* New York: Routledge, 2008.

18. James Byrne, "Press Release: *Eyes Wide Open.*" New York: Dance Theater Workshop (20 April 1989), 1.

19. Amy Greenfield, "Introduction." *Filmdance 1890s–1983.* New York: Exhibition catalog.

20. See for example: Judy Mitoma, *Envisioning Dance on Film and Video* (New York: Routledge, 2002).

21. The International Screendance Network is a group of US- and UK-based researchers and practitioners established to advance an interdisciplinary, theoretical, and practice-based discourse on screendance. Members include Claudia Kappenberg (Principal Investigator, University of Brighton), Sarah Whatley (Co-Investigator, Coventry University) Douglas Rosenberg (University of Wisconsin-Madison), Marisa Zanotti (Chichester University), Ann Cooper Albright (Oberlin College, Ohio), Simon Ellis (Roehampton University, UK) and Harmony Bench (Ohio State University). Past members: Katrina McPherson (choreographer/video dance-maker/producer) and Christinn Whyte (Middlesex University, freelance writer).

22. André Bazin, *What is Cinema?*, vol. 1, trans. Hugh Gray (Berkeley: University of California Press, 1967), 21.

23. *Screendance Has Not Yet Been Invented* became the title of the first issue of *The International Journal of Screendance* published by Parallel Press, University of Wisconsin-Madison, http://journals.library.wisc.edu/index.php/screendance (Douglas Rosenberg, Claudia Kappenberg, editors) as well as a part of the critical framework of The International Screendance Network Symposium in Brighton, 2011.

8 "SEEING IS FORGETTING THE NAME OF THE THING ONE SEES OR CONNOISSEURSHIP IN SCREENDANCE

1. Lawrence Weschler, *Seeing is Forgetting the Name of the Thing One Sees*, (Los Angeles: University of California Press).

2. Susan Sontag, *On Photography* (New York: Picador, 1973), 116.

3. The crisis of identity that screendance suffers, (see chap. xxx) is shared by audiences as well. On a spectrum of art and entertainment, screendance is initiated with multiple intentionalities and subsequent outcomes, and audiences often attend festival screenings and other exhibitions with competing desires, in part resulting from the plethora of genres and styles grouped together at most screendance festivals. Further complicating this is the way in which artworks at the intersection of dance and media are described: "screendance," "dance film" and "video dance" all imply a unique relationship between distinct practices, which if correctly applied, have particularity and specificity. Additionally, there is a lack of

attention to genre and curatorial rigor on the part of institutions that disseminate and present screendance. See also Rosenberg, "Curating the Practice/The
Practice of Curating," *International Journal of Performance Arts and Digital Media*
5 (December 2009): 75–87.

4. Noël Carroll, *Engaging the Moving Image* (New Haven, CT: Yale University Press,
2003), 133.

5. Elizabeth Ezra, *George Méliès: The Birth of the Auteur* (New York: Manchester
University Press, 2000), 17.

6. Chirstinn Whyte, "The Evolution of the 'A' Word, Changing Notions of Professional
Practice in Avant-Garde Film and Contemporary Screendance" *International
Journal of Screendance* 1 (Summer 2010): 7–12, quotation on 7.

7. Patrick Phillips, "Spectator, audience and response," in *An Introduction to Film
Studies*, ed. Jill Nelmes (New York: Routledge, 1996), 94.

8. Ibid.

9. Mark K. Smith, "Elliot W. Eisner, connoisseurship, criticism and the art of education," in *The Encyclopaedia of Informal Education,* 2005. Web. 12 July 2010.

10. Ibid.

11. Tamara Harvey, "'What About the Audience?/What About Them?': Spectatorship
and Cinematic Pleasure," *Paroles Gelées* 14.2 (1996): 154.

12. Michele Aaron, *Spectatorship: The Power of Looking On* (London: Wallflower Press,
2007), 16.

13. Quoted in Smith, "Elliot W. Eisner," Web.

14. Phillips, "Spectator, audience and response," 94.

15. Barbara Newsom and Adele Silver, eds. *The Art Museum as Educator: A Collection of
Studies as Guides to Practice and Policy* (New York: University of California Press,
1978).

16. Quoted. in Douglas Crimp, "The Photographic Activity of Postmodernism," in
Postmodernism: A Reader, ed. Thomas Docherty (New York: Columbia University
Press, 1993), 176.

17. Ibid. Both artists and critics in this case are aware of Walter Benjamin's theories
about mechanical reproduction and the diminishment of the value of the
original via its copies. Rose names mechanical reproduction and more specifically
photography as the oppositional force in the kind of painting she describes.

18. Douglas Crimp, "Pictures," *October* 8 (Spring 1979): 75–88.

19. Crimp, "Photographic Activity," 176.

20. Ibid.

21. See press release titled "Dance Camera West Presents 'Body/Traces,' a Site-Specific
Media Installation During Downtown Los Angeles Art Walk." 1 June 2010. Web
Retrieved 8 August, 2010 from: http://www.dancecamerawest.org/2010_DCW_
PR2.html

22. Kate Mondloch, *Screens: Viewing Media Installation Art* (Minneapolis: University
of Minnesota Press, 2010), 25–26.

23. Michael Brenson, *Acts of Engagement: Writings on Art, Criticism, and Institutions, 1993–2002* (New York: Rowman and Littlefield Publishers, Inc., 2004),
40–41.

9 TOWARD A THEORY OF SCREENDANCE

1. Here I hope to shift the discourse from distribution platforms to one that engages
the critical apparatus of the field in order to clarify and focus an evolving theory
of screendance.

2. For more of Lepecki's ideas about contemporary dance, see *Exhausting Dance: Performance and the Politics of Movement* (New York: Routledge, 2006).

3. Sally Banes, and Noël Carroll, "Cunningham, Balanchine, and Postmodern Dance, *Dance Chronicle* 29 (2006): 49–68, quotation on 51.

4. Arthur C. Danto, *After the End of Art: Contemporary Art and the Pale of History,* (Princeton, NJ: Princeton University Press, 1998), 137.

5. Karen Pearlman, "Crossing the Divide," *RealTime+OnScreen* 78 (April–May 2007): 31. Web. 5 Sep 2009.

6. See Maurice Merleau-Ponty, *Phenomenology of Perception* (New York: Routledge Classics, 2002).

7. Susan Manning, *Modern Dance, Negro Dance: Race in Motion* (Minneapolis: University of Minnesota Press, 2004), xix.

8. For an examination of the relationship between bodies in motion and projected media, see Mark Boucher, "Kinetic Synaesthesia: Experiencing Dance in Multimedia Scenographies," *Contemporary Aesthetics*. Web. 15 May 2011.

9. Laura Mulvey, "Visual Pleasure and Narrative Cinema," *Screen* 16.3 (Autumn 1975): 6–18.

10. Ibid.

11. Peggy Phelan, "Preface: Arresting Performances of Sexual and Racial Difference: Toward a Theory of Performative Film," *Women & Performance: A Journal of Feminist Theory* 6.2 (1993): 5–10, quotation on 7.

12. Amy Greenfield, "The Kinesthetics of Avant-Garde Dance Film: Deren and Harris," in *Envisioning Dance on Film and Video*, ed. Judy Mitoma, Elizabeth Zimmer, and Dale Ann Stieber (New York: Routledge, 2002), 21–26.

13. "New Television Workshop." *WGBH*. Web. 9 Oct 2010.

14. Greenfield, "Kinesthetics of Avant-Garde Dance Film," 26.

15. For a complete reading of Greenfield's text on the film I recommend her chapter in Mitoma et al., *Envisioning Dance*.

16. Greenfield, "Kinesthetics of Avant-Garde Dance Film," 24.

17. Ibid., 24.

18. Ibid., 25.

19. See Noël Carroll, *A Philosophy of Mass Art* (Oxford: Oxford University Press, 1998).

20. See for instance Richard Schechner, *The Future of Ritual: Writings on Culture and Performance* (New York: Routledge, 1993).

21. *Screening the Body: Tracing Medicine's Visual Culture*. Minneapolis: University of Minnesota Press, 1995. xi–xii. Print.

22. Ibid., 3.

10 NEGOTIATING THE ACADEMY

1. The University of Brighton offers a master of arts degree in Performance and Visual Practice and the University of Utah offers a graduate certificate in screendance.

2. Diana Burgess Fuller and Daniela Salvioni, eds., *Art/Women/California, 1950–2000: Parallels and Intersections* (Berkeley: University of California Press, 2002), 317.

3. See chap. 4 for an outline of video's interdisciplinary roots. To reiterate a quotation from that chapter: "Video's pedigree is anything but pure. Conceived from a promiscuous mix of disciplines in the great optimism of post–World War II culture, its stock of practitioners includes a jumble of musicians, poets, documentarians, sculptors, painters, dancers and technology freaks. Its lineage can be traced

to the discourses of art, science, linguistics, technology, mass media, and politics. Cutting across such diverse fields, early video displays a broad range of concerns, often linked by nothing more than the tools themselves. Nonetheless, the challenge of video's history has been taken on by the art world, though it might well have been claimed by social history or, for that matter, the history of science and technology. Art historians, however, face two obstacles to constructing a credible history of video: video's multiple origins and its explicitly anti-establishment beginnings." Doug Hall and Sally Jo Feiffer, *Illuminating Video: An Essential Guide to Video Art* (Ann Arbor: University of Michigan Press, 1990), 14.

4. Screendance, with a similar history and as a subgenre of video art, would fare equally well if sited in a similarly interdisciplinary milieu. In the case of screendance, it would also seem logical that dance be a part of the interdisciplinary partnership along with video art, theory, and other such appropriate disciplines.

5. I use the term "video" to denote a historical frame while acknowledging that the term is a fluid one. Video is a porous boundary that includes digital media as well.

6. David Hall, "Early Video Art: A Look at a Controversial History," in *Diverse Practices*, ed. Julia Knight. (Luton, UK: John Libbey Media, 1996), 71–80, quotation on 76.

7. I have relied on, among others, Walter Benjamin's theories about mechanical reproduction, Lucy Lippard's theories about the dematerialization of the body, and Phillip Auslander's writings about liveness as examples of scholarship that are parallel to the concerns of screendance.

8. This includes such events as Open Source VideoDance in Scotland, the publication of the first *International Journal of Screendance*, The Screendance Network and other such endeavors.

9. "Converge: Works by Ana Mendieta and Hans Breder, 1970–1980," *Oneartworld. com*. Web. 10 Oct 2010.

10. Elaine Summers, "Infinite Choices," in *Intermedia: Enacting the Liminal*, ed. Hans Breder and Klaus-Peter Busse (Dortmund, Germany: Dortmunder Schriften zur Kunst. 197–202), 200.

11. Claudia Tatinge Nascimento, "A Tri-dimensional Mapping of the Field," *Dance Research Journal* 32.1 (Summer, 2000): 165–67, quotation on 165.

12. See Henry Sayre, *The Object of Performance* (Chicago: University of Chicago Press, 1992).

SELECTED BIBLIOGRAPHY

Aaron, Michele. *Spectatorship: The Power of Looking On*. London: Wallflower Press, 2007.

Adorno, Theodor. *The Culture Industry*. New York: Routledge, 2001.

Anderson, Benedict. *Imagined Communities*. New York: Verso, 1983.

Arlen, Michael. *Living-Room War*. Syracuse: Syracuse University Press, 1997.

Ascott, Roy. "Is There Love in the Telematic Embrace?" *Art Journal* 49.3 (1990): 241–47.

Auslander, Phillip. *Liveness: Performance in a Mediatized Culture*. New York: Routledge, 1999.

Baldwin, Neil. *Edison: Inventing the Century*. New York: Hyperion, 1995.

Banes, Sally, and Noël Carroll. "Cunningham, Balanchine, and Postmodern Dance." *Dance Chronicle* 29 (2006): 49–68.

Banes, Sally. *Dancing Women: Female Bodies on Stage*. New York: Routledge, 1998.

———. *Terpsichore in Sneakers*. Hanover, NH: University Press of New England, 1987.

———. *Writing Dancing in the Age of Postmodernism*. Middletown, CT: Wesleyan University Press, 1994.

Barthes, Roland. *Camera Lucida: Reflections on Photography*. Translated by Richard Howard. New York: Hill and Wang, 1981.

———. *Roland Barthes*. Translated by Richard Howard. London: Macmillan, 1977.

Bazin, André. *What is Cinema?* Vol. 1. Translated by Hugh Gray. Berkeley: University of California Press, 1967.

Benjamin, Walter. "The Work of Art in The Age of Mechanical Reproduction." In *Modern Art and Modernism: A Critical Anthology*, edited by Francis Frascina and Charles Harrison, 217–27. New York: The Open University, 1982.

———. *Reflections: Essays, Aphorisms, Autobiographical Writings*. Edited by Peter Demetz. New York: Schocken Books, Inc.

Berger, John. *About Looking*. New York: Pantheon Books, 1980.

Boucher, Mark. "Kinetic Synaesthesia: Experiencing Dance in Multimedia Scenographies." Contemporary Aesthetics. Web. http://www.contempaesthetics.org/newvolume/pages/article.php?articleID=235. 15 May 2011.

Brannigan, Erin. "Modern Movement, Dance, and the Birth of Cinema." In *Dancefilm: Choreography and the Moving Image*, 19–38. Oxford: Oxford University Press, 2011.

———. "Yvonne Rainer." *Senses of Cinema* 27 (2003). Web. http://www.sensesofcinema.com/2003/great-directors/rainer/. 18 November 2007.

Brenson, Michael. *Acts of Engagement: Writings on Art, Criticism, and Institutions, "1993–2002*. New York: Rowman and Littlefield Publishers, Inc., 2004.

Brooks, Virginia. "From Méliès to Streaming Video: A Century of Moving Dance Images." In *Envisioning Dance on Film and Video*, edited by Judy Mitoma, 54–60. New York: Routledge, 2002.

Burris, Jon. "Did the Portapak Cause Video Art? Notes On the Formation of a New Medium." *Millennium Film Journal* 29 (1996): 3–28.

Bush, Jeffrey, and Peter Z. Grossman. "Videodance." *DanceScope* 9, no. 2 (1975): 12–17.

Byrne, James. "Press Release: *Eyes Wide Open.*" New York: Dance Theater Workshop. April 20, 1989: 1.

Carroll, Noël. *On Criticism*. New York: Routledge, 2009.

———. *A Philosophy of Mass Art*. New York: Oxford University Press, 1998.

———. "Toward a Definition of Moving-Picture Dance." In *Engaging the Moving Image*, 234–54. New Haven, CT: Yale University Press, 2003.

Cartwright, Lisa. *Screening the Body: Tracing Medicine's Visual Culture*. Minneapolis: University of Minnesota Press, 1995.

Caws, Mary Ann, ed. *Manifesto: A Century of Isms*. Lincoln: University of Nebraska Press, 2000.

Clark, Ronald W. *Edison: The Man Who Made the Future*. New York: G. P. Putnam's Sons, 1977.

Clegg, Brian. *The Man Who Stopped Time: The Illuminating Story of Eadweard Muybridge: Pioneer Photographer, Father of the Motion Picture, Murderer*. Washington, DC: Joseph Henry Press, 2007.

Copeland, Roger. "Merce Cunningham and the Politics of Perception." In *What is Dance? Readings in Theory and Criticism*, edited by Roger Copeland and Marshall Cohen, 307–24. London: Oxford University Press, 1983.

———. *The Modernizing of Modern Dance*. New York: Routledge, 2004.

Cox, Geoff, and Joasia Krysa. "O zadaniach kuratorw wobec obiektw niematerialnych: generowanie I uszkadzanie obiektw cyfrowych" (Immaterial Curating: the generation and corruption of the digital object). Translated by Marta Walkowiak. In *Zeszyty Artystyczne*, edited by Lukasz Ronduda, 104–15. Poznan: Uniwersytet Poznanski, 2003.

Crimp, Douglas. "The Photographic Activity of Postmodernism." In *Postmodernism: A Reader*, edited by Thomas Docherty, 172–79. New York: Columbia University Press, 1993.

———. "Pictures." *October* 8 (1979): 75–88.

Danto, Arthur C. *After the End of Art: Contemporary Art and the Pale of History*. Princeton, NJ: Princeton University Press, 1998.

Decker-Phillips, Edith. *Paik Video*. Barrytown, NY: Barrytown LTD, 1998.

Deren, Maya. *An Anagram of Ideas on Art, Form and Film*. Yonkers, NY: The Alicat Book Shop Press, 1946.

Derrida, Jacques. *Archive Fever: A Freudian Impression*. Translated by Eric Prenowitz. Chicago: University of Chicago Press, 1995.

Dodds, Sherril. *Dance on Screen: Genres and Media from Hollywood to Experimental Art*. New York: Palgrave, 2001.

The Drama Review 19.1–4 (1975).

Ezra, Elizabeth. *George Méliès: The Birth of the Auteur*. Manchester: Manchester University Press, 2000.

Falco, Charles M. "Use of Optics by Renaissance Artists." *McGraw Hill AccessScience: Encyclopedia of Science and Technology Online*. Web. 20 March 2010.

Federman, Mark. "What is the Meaning of the Medium is the Message?" Web. 4 January 2010.

Foster, Hal. *The Return of the Real: The Avant-Garde at the End of the Century*. Cambridge, MA: MIT Press, 1996.

Franko, Mark. "Aesthetic Agencies in Flux." In *Maya Deren and the American Avant-Garde*, edited by Bill Nichols, 131–50. Berkeley: University of California Press, 2001.

Fuller, Diana Burgess, and Daniela Salvioni, eds. *Art/Women/California, 1950–2000: Parallels and Intersections*. Berkeley: University of California Press, 2002.

Giesen, Bernhard. "Performance Art." *Social Performance: Symbolic Action, Cultural Pragmatics, and Ritual*, edited by Jeffrey C. Alexander, Bernhard Giesen, and Jason L. Mast, 315–24. Cambridge: Cambridge University Press, 2006.

Glass, Philip. "Photographer." *New York Times*, 7 October 1983. Web. 15 April 2011.

Goldberg, Rose Lee. *Performance: Live Art: 1909 to the Present*. Ann Arbor: University of Michigan Press, 1979.

Greenfield, Amy. "The Kinesthetics of Avant-Garde Dance Film: Deren and Harris." In *Envisioning Dance on Film and Video*, edited by Judy Mitoma, Elizabeth Zimmer, and Dale Ann Stieber, 21–26. New York: Routledge, 2002.

———. "Dance as Film." *Filmmakers Newsletter* 4.1 (1970): 26.

Gunning, Tom. "Chaplin and the Body of Modernity." *Proceedings of The BFI Charles Chaplin Conference, July 2005*. Web. 13 March 2011.

Hall, David. "Early Video Art: A Look at a Controversial History." In *Diverse Practices*, edited by Julia Knight, 71–80. Luton, UK: John Libbey Media, 1996.

Hall, Doug, and Sally Jo Feiffer. *Illuminating Video: An Essential Guide to Video Art*. Ann Arbor: University of Michigan Press, 1990.

Harvey, Tamara. "'What About the Audience?/What About Them?': Spectatorship and Cinematic Pleasure." *Paroles Gelées* 14.2 (1996): 153–62.

Hayles, N. Katherine. "Print Is Flat, Code Is Deep: The Importance of Media-Specific Analysis." *Poetics Today* 25.1 (2004): 67–90.

Hayward, Susan. *Cinema Studies: The Key Concepts*. 2nd ed. New York: Routledge, 2000.

Hendricks, Gordon. *Eadweard Muybridge: The Father of the Motion Picture*. London: Secker and Warburg, 1975.

Hjort, Mette, and Scott MacKenzie, eds. *Purity and Provocation: Dogma 95*. London: British Film Institute, 2003.

Jameson, Frederick. *Postmodernism, or, The Cultural Logic of Late Capitalism*. Durham: Duke University Press, 1991.

Jones, Amelia. "'Presence' in Absentia: Experiencing Performance as Documentation." *Art Journal* 56.4 (1997): 11–18.

Josephson, Matthew. *Edison: A Biography*. New York: McGraw-Hill, 1959.

Kappenberg, Claudia. "Does Screendance Need to Look like Dance?" *International Journal of Performance Arts and Digital Media* 5.2–3 (2009): 89–105.

Kaprow, Allan. *Essays on the Blurring of Art and Life*. Rev. ed. Edited by Jeff Kelley. Los Angeles: University of California Press, 2003.

Kearns, Mary Ann. "The Role of Technology in the Art of Nam June Paik: Paik's Videotapes." The Experimental Television Center's Video History Project. 1988. Web. 11 November 2010.

Kelley, Jeff. *Childsplay: The Art of Allan Kaprow*. Berkeley: University of California Press, 2004.

Kepes, Gyorgy. *The Visual Arts Today*. Middletown, CT: Wesleyan University Press, 1960.

Kisselgoff, Anna. "Dance: Joanne Kelley With Tape." *New York Times*, 20 November 1977: 67.

Krauss, Rosalind. "Video: The Esthetics of Narcissism." *October* 1 (1976): 50–64.

Kwon, Miwon. *One Place After Another: Site-Specific Art and Locational Identity*. Cambridge, MA: MIT Press, 2004.

Lepecki, Andre. *Exhausting Dance: Performance and the Politics of Movement*. New York: Routledge, 2006.

Lippard, Lucy. *Six Years: The Dematerialization of the Art Object from 1966 to 1972*. Los Angeles: University of California Press, 1997.

Lippit, Akira Mizuta. *Migrations of Gesture*. Minneapolis: University of Minnesota Press, 2008.

Lovejoy, Margot. *Postmodern Currents: Art and Artists in the Age of Electronic Media*. 2nd ed. Upper Saddle River, NJ: Prentice Hall, 1997.

MacDonnell, Kevin. *Eadweard Muybridge: The Man Who Invented the Moving Picture*. London: Weidenfield and Nicolson, 1972.

Manning, Susan. *Modern Dance, Negro Dance: Race in Motion*. Minneapolis: University of Minnesota Press, 2004.

Manovich, Lev. *The Language of New Media*. Boston: MIT Press, 2002.

Martin, John Joseph. *John Martin's Book of the Dance*. New York: Tudor, 1963.

McCarren, Felicia M. "The Dancer, the Train, and the Cinema." In *Dancing Machines: Choreographies in the Age of Mechanical Reproduction*, 43–44. Stanford, CA: Stanford University Press, 2003.

McLuhan, Marshall. "The Medium Is the Message." In *Essential McLuhan*, edited by Eric McLuhan and Frank Zingrone. New York: Basic Books, 1995.

McPherson, Katrina, Litza Bixler and Deveril. "Dogma Dance." *left-luggage.co.uk*. 18 August 2007. Web. 12 March 2010.

Merleau-Ponty, Maurice. *Phenomenology of Perception*. New York: Routledge Classics, 2002.

Mitoma, Judy, ed. *Envisioning Dance on Film and Video*. New York: Routledge, 2002.

Mitra, Ananda, and Rae Lynn Schwartz. "From Cyber Space to Cybernetic Space: Rethinking the Relationship between Real and Virtual Spaces." *Journal of Computer-Mediated Communication* 7.1 (2001). Web. 1 May 2011.

Mondloch, Kate. *Screens: Viewing Media Installation Art*. Minneapolis: University of Minnesota Press, 2010.

Mulvey, Laura. "Visual Pleasure and Narrative Cinema." *Screen* 16.3 (1975): 6–18.

Musser, Charles. "At the Beginning: Motion Picture Production, Representation and Ideology at the Edison and Lumière companies." In *The Silent Cinema Reader*, edited by. Lee Grieveson and Peter Krämer. New York: Routledge, 2004.

Nascimento, Claudia Tatinge. "A Tri-dimensional Mapping of the Field." *Dance Research Journal* 32.1 (2000): 165–67.

Nelmes, Jill, ed. *An Introduction to Film Studies*. New York: Routledge, 1996.

Ness, Sally Ann. "The Inscription of Gesture: Inward Migrations in Dance." In *Migrations of Gesture*, edited by Carrie Noland and Sally Ann Ness, 1–30. Minneapolis: University of Minnesota Press, 2008.

Newsom, Barbara, and Adele Silver, eds. *The Art Museum as Educator: A Collection of Studies as Guides to Practice and Policy*. New York: University of California Press, 1978.

O'Neill, Paul. "The Curatorial Turn: From Practice to Discourse." In *Issues in Curating Contemporary Art and Performance*, edited by Judith Rugg and Michele Sedgwick, 14–15. Chicago: Chicago University Press, 2008.

Pearlman, Karen. "Crossing the Divide." *RealTime+OnScreen* 78 (2007). Web. 5 Sep 2009.

Peterson, Sidney. *The Avant-Garde Film: A Reader of Theory and Practice*. Edited by P. Adams Sitney. New York: New York University Press, 1978.

Phelan, Peggy. "Preface: Arresting Performances of Sexual and Racial Difference: Toward a Theory of Performative Film." *Women & Performance: A Journal of Feminist Theory* 6.2 (1993): 5–10.

Poster, Mark, ed. *Jean Baudrillard, Selected Writings*. Stanford: Stanford University Press, 1988.

Rainer, Yvonne. "Some Retrospective Notes on a Dance for 10 People and 12 Mattresses Called Parts of Some Sextets." In *Happenings and Other Acts,* edited by Mariellen R. Sandford, 130–37. London: Routledge, 1995.

Reason, Matthew, and Dee Reynolds. "Special Issue Editorial: Screen Dance Audiences—Why Now?" *Journal of Audience and Reception Studies* 7.2 (2010). Web. 24 February 2011.

Rosenberg, Douglas. "Video Space: A Site for Choreography." *LEONARDO: Journal of the International Society for the Arts, Sciences and Technology* 33.4 (2000): 275–80.

Rush, Michael. *New Media in Late 20th-Century Art*. London: Thames and Hudson, 1999.

Sayre, Henry M. *The Object of Performance: The American Avant-Garde since 1970*. Chicago: University of Chicago Press, 1989.

Schechner, Richard. *The Future of Ritual: Writings on Culture and Performance*. New York: Routledge, 1993.

———. *Performance Theory*. Rev. ed. New York: Routledge, 1988.

Silverman, Lois H. "Making Meaning Together: Lessons from the field of American History." In *Reinventing the Museum: Historical and Contemporary Perspectives on the Paradigm Shift,* edited by Gail Anderson, 233–42. Oxford: Roman and Littlefield Publishers, Inc., 2004.

Smith, Mark K. "Elliot W. Eisner, Connoisseurship, Criticism and the Art of Education." *The Encyclopaedia of Informal Education*. 2005. Web. 12 July 2010.

Solnit, Rebecca. *River of Shadows: Eadweard Muybridge and the Technological Wild West*. New York: Viking, 2003.

Solomon, Larry J. "The Sounds of Silence: John Cage and 4'33"." *Media Art Net*. 2002. Web. 15 October 2010.

Sontag, Susan. *Against Interpretation and Other Essays*. New York: Picador, 1966.

———. *On Photography*. New York: Anchor Books/Doubleday, 1989.

Stoos, Toni, and Thomas Kellein, eds. *Nam June Paik: Video Time, Video Space*. New York: H. N. Abrams, 1998.

Suchenski, Richard. "Hans Richter." *Senses of Cinema*. Web. 15 March 2010.

Summers, Elaine. "Infinite Choices." In *Intermedia: Enacting the Liminal,* edited by Hans Breder and Klaus-Peter Busse, 197–202. Germany: Dortmunder Schriften zur Kunst, 2005.

Theall, Donald F., and Edmund Carpenter. *The Virtual Marshall McLuhan*. Montreal: McGill-Queen's University Press, 2001.

Tomkins, Calvin. *Duchamp: A Biography*. New York: Henry Holt and Company, Inc., 1996.

Vaughan, David. "Locale: The Collaboration of Merce Cunningham and Charles Atlas." *Millennium Film Journal* 10/11 (1981–82): 18–22.

Wells, Liz. "Curatorial Strategy as Critical Intervention: The Genesis of Facing East." In Rugg and Sedgwick, *Issues in Curating Contemporary Art and Performance*, 29–45.

Weschler, Lawrence. *Seeing is Forgetting the Name of the Thing One Sees*. Berkeley: University of California Press, 1982.

Whyte, Chirstinn. "The Evolution of the 'A' Word, Changing Notions of Professional Practice in Avant-Garde Film and Contemporary Screendance." *International Journal of Screendance* 1 (2010): 7–12.

INDEX

Cunningham, Merce, 47, 80, 88, 143, 156
    Blue Studio: Five Segments, 87–88, 164
    John Cage, work with, 97
    Locale, 30–31, 32f
    Nam June Paik, work with, 85
curating screendance, 126–140
    criticality and, 10, 127–128
    curatorial activism, lack of, 5
    curators, role of, 130, 137
    importance of, 139–140
    statements, 135–136
"The Curatorial Turn: From Practice to Discourse" (O'Neill), 129–130
curriculum, screendance, 176. *see also* courses, screendance

Dada movement, 51, 58, 67, 82, 121, 168
Dali, Salvador, 42
dance
    "dance by the camera," 26–27
    "dance on film" festivals, 144
    discipline of, 171
    documentation, 18–28, 64–65
    ephemeral nature of, 14
    genres of, 112, 116
    history, 33–35
    indexes of, 34
    language of, 110, 112, 155–156
    live performances, 7, 22–23, 102–104
    media and, 1–2, 11, 120, 126–127
    moving images and, 6–7, 159
    screendance, relationship to, 4, 158, 176–177
    technology and, 93–109
    for television, 20–21, 183n8
    theory, 177
"Dance as Film" (Greenfield), 7
dance for camera, 15, 16, 18, 113–114
    Dance for Camera conference, 179
    defined, 3
"Dance in America," 72
A Dance in the Sun (Clarke), 86–87
Dance on Screen: Genres and Media from Hollywood to Experimental Art (Dodds), 20–21, 34, 111–112, 127
Dance Theater Workshop (DTW), 133, 135

Dancefilm, Choreography and the Moving Image (Brannigan), 127
Dancing Girl: A Pirouette (Muybridge), 37f
Dancing Girl. A Pirouette. From Animal Locomotion: An Electro-Photographic Investigation of Consecutive Phases of Animal Movement (1872–1885) (Muybridge), 56f
Danto, Arthur, 157
De Jong, Bettie, 65–68, 165–167
De Keersmaeker, Anne Teresa, 88
    Rosas Danst Rosas, 11, 162f, 164–165, 168
De Mey, Thierry
    One Flat Thing, Reproduced, 164
    Rosas Danst Rosas, 164–165, 168
Decker-Phillips, Edith, 83
Decoufle, Phillipe, 164
Dendy, Mark, 170
Deren, Maya, 2, 12
    amateurism, 143
    cine-dance, work in, 8
    experimental film, work in, 137, 177
    film dance, definition of, 119–120
    on historical continuum of dance on screen, 34–35
    influences on, 42–43
    Meshes of the Afternoon, 42
    A Study in Choreography for Camera, 6, 41–43, 48–50, 65, 87, 98, 167
    Witch's Cradle, 47
Derrida, Jacques, 156
    Archive Fever, A Freudian Impression, 25–26
desires, competing, 143, 149, 152
Deveril, 118
Di Maria, Walter, Lightning Field, 78
dialectic of dance and media, 120
difference, articulation of, 151
"Digesture" (Lippit), 55
digital culture, tensions of, 104
digital technology
    editing, 68
    video, 21–22
digressive moments in film, 43–44, 46
directors, 159–160
Dirt (Greenfield), 134
disciplines, academic, 110, 117, 171–173, 175–176. *see also* interdisciplinarity